P9-DKE-843

Praise for *The Pain-Free Back*

**Easy-to-follow exercises make this an invaluable book for those who seek a path to healing.**

"Back pain is a common occurrence that frustrates and limits many people. It can be extremely debilitating, with causes that are not always understood and treatments that are often not effective. In *The Pain-Free Back: 54 Simple Qigong Movements for Healing and Prevention*, Dr. Yang, Jwing-Ming shares information on the causes and treatments of back pain from both Western and Eastern perspectives as well as a series of exercises to improve back function and eliminate pain through the manipulation of qi.

"The book starts with a fascinating explanation of the Chinese approach to medicine and to back pain specifically. This is a general introduction that will be new to many Westerners, and it offers unique insight into the concept of health and well-being in Chinese culture. The book then goes into the various causes of back pain, compares how the Chinese address back pain with how it is treated in the West, and explains how qigong can be used to treat back pain. After describing the various exercises, it concludes with a glossary of Chinese terms and an extensive list of the author's other publications.

"Perhaps because the spine is central to all of the functions of the human body, this book shares information on qigong practice that is incredibly complex, with details about the eight vessels and the twelve channels through which qi moves and about the anatomical structure of the back and spine. There is also a brief explanation of how the central nervous system functions. Though this material is a little intimidating, Yang's explanations are very straightforward, and the information is necessary to understand how and why the suggested exercises work.

"The exercises offered here are gentle and intended to be done with mindfulness and while relaxed. The author explains

"'Qigong teaches you how to regulate the mind to a calm, profound, and concentrated meditative state. It also teaches you how to use your regulated mind in coordination with deep breathing to lead the qi circulating in your body.'

"This practice is bound to appeal to those who live with pain. The exercises are carefully and thoroughly explained; black-and-white photographs show each motion, with helpful arrows illustrating how to move.

"*The Pain-Free Back* offers hope for relief to anyone who has ever suffered from back pain. The straightforward yet thoughtful presentation of information, coupled with easy-to-follow exercises, makes this an invaluable book for those who seek a path to healing beyond what standard Western therapies have to offer. It also serves as a solid introduction to qigong practice, which may be helpful in others aspects of healing."
—Catherine Thureson, *Foreword Reviews*

"If you want to resolve chronic back pain, you need to heal the spine and rebuild its strength. In this masterful volume of qigong exercises, Dr. Yang, Jwing-Ming shows you how to achieve positive results within just three months."
—Dr. Mark Wiley, MS, OMD, PhD; contributor, EasyHealthOptions.com; publisher, Tambuli Media

"As an expert on the resolution of back pain, I was flattered at the opportunity to lend my endorsement to Dr. Yang, Jwing-Ming's latest work. This book is comprehensive and very engaging, starting with a thorough overview of Western medical approaches to the treatment of back pain as a basis for understanding and appreciating Dr. Yang's more traditional qigong methods. Dr. Yang offers timely and respectful alternatives to the conventional Western medical approach, using qigong as a way to resolve or avoid back pain outright. His practical self-care resources make for an effective blending of ancient wisdom and modern medicine that any reader can apply at home on their own. Another home run for Dr. Yang."

—John Loupos, MS, HSE, author of *The Sustainable You: Somatics and the Myth of Aging* and *Tai Chi Connections: Advancing Your Tai Chi Experience*; owner of the Pain and Mobility Clinic, Cohasset, Massachusetts

"Dr. Yang presents an informative and helpful approach to the management of back pain in an easy-to-understand format. Providing a layout of the anatomy of the spine as well as several possibilities of the causes of back pain will allow the reader to feel empowered and knowledgeable. As a classical Pilates instructor, I especially appreciate the exercises being broken down into categories for stretching, strengthening, and pain relief. This will give readers options depending on what their needs are at any given time and help the book to stay relevant and useful indefinitely."

—Sally Whitaker, Peak Pilates comprehensive instructor; studio manager at Studio on Main Pilates & Yoga, Independence, Missouri; owner of Move Forward Pilates

# Testimonials

Having a healthy back, in my case, truly required committing myself to a healthy way of life. Central to this healthy way of life has been my study of martial arts for the past twenty-three years—the last six years of which I have pursued under the guidance of Master Yang.

Many of you who read this will be able to prevent or cure back problems by simple, regular practice of the movements and methods contained in this book. Some of you may need to go much deeper as I have needed to and solve the inner mysteries that have led to your back problems. In either case, I believe all will benefit, as I have, with regular practice of these time-tested techniques.

In my life, my poor health manifested most intensely through severe, debilitating pain in my lower back. I was often completely incapacitated during my teens and early adulthood. My suffering can be traced back to a severe injury when I was six years old. I had my toes cut off of my left foot and surgically reattached. Subsequently, my functionally "club" foot distorted my whole skeletal growth through my formative years. By the age of twenty-one, I was told by prominent medical doctors that I had the "spine of a senior citizen," I would "never be a carpenter," I would never have a job that involved standing on my feet, I would "never be a gymnast," and that I "ought to get a desk job." From the perspective of eliminating pain, traditional medicine could offer only drugs and surgery. I did not feel I could restore my health following this path.

Fortunately, I had been training in the martial arts for three years, and I had glimpsed a ray of hope. Although the knowledge I was exposed to was only superficial relative to the knowledge

Dr. Yang shares, I was on "The Way." Along "The Way" I found adjunctive healing modalities helpful in the development of a strong core and spinal health. Chiropractic acupuncture, various massage forms, dietary changes, and graduate studies in holistic education and counseling have been major players in my health prescription. Again, central to these healing methods was my internal development, mainly due to my daily martial arts practice. For many years I was training just to avoid pain and, depending on these "alternative" therapies, to straighten me out when I erred. Gradually, as my practice moved me toward health rather than just away from illness, my dependence on external therapies for alleviation of pain virtually ceased. Now, I can use these healing tools on occasion to prevent problems and increase my health.

The techniques described in this book can be made central or adjunctive to your healing process. Either way, it is important to take note of the major themes in this book. Not only are they central to the traditional martial arts, but they are also a core part of any health prescription. These themes include taking responsibility for your life, taking a leap of faith (though not blind faith) in the healing process, learning to accept life's difficulties, and fully committing to the process of learning and healing.

If "age is the condition of the spine" (a yogic belief), then a painful spine is an old spine. It is diseased, not at ease. Regular practice of the movements described in this book in a relaxed, centered, and grounded manner will help guide you out of dis-ease and into ease; improve the condition of your spine; bring a loving, youthful bounce back to your step; and help you to understand yourself and life's mysteries. I know this to be true.

**Roger Whidden**
**Martial arts teacher**

Three days before my college graduation, I had the misfortune to be a passenger in a Subaru that broadsided a Lincoln Continental. At the hospital, the doctor asked me what I did for my scoliosis. "What scoliosis?" I asked, unsure whether it was a spine or a liver problem. "This one," he said, holding up an X-ray that looked more like a roller coaster than a spine.

Up to that point, I had had no problems with my back. I trained in karate and gongfu, and though my left side kick and right front kick wobbled when thrown, I always assumed it had something to do with laziness. In the back of my head, I had wondered why I could do the splits but not touch my toes. But, like many other twenty-two-year-olds, I moved on to other thoughts rather than resolve those.

After the accident, I spent nearly two years trying to contain a constant, severe ache. Doctors recommended nautilus and walking. Chiropractors shrugged and apologized. Two years after the accident, I returned to taiji. I also got Rolfed. Now when I practiced diligently, I could have pain-free days if I didn't stress my back. The problem with this situation was that I owned an ice-cream truck business. If you have never had the pleasure, let me tell you that being and ice-cream truck driver, and especially knowing other ice-cream truck drivers, can really stress your back. So, I resigned myself to low-level pain.

By 1990, I was out of the ice-cream truck and in an office. I practiced my form regularly and had contained my back problems. It ached when I was tired, stressed, or physically active, but I was prepared to live with that.

Then, in August 1990, I stopped by the YMAA school just to take a look. From the first warm-up exercises, I saw a new path. Spine loosening and flexing is a focal point of all of the training. It takes years to begin to understand how to move the spine, how to relax the joints and the muscles in and around the spine. The process opened my eyes. Although over the years I had bored many a friend with discussions about back pain (have you ever been in an interesting one?), I didn't know my back. I didn't know how to move individual pieces and relax individual muscles.

The health benefits associated with learning to move this way are enormous. I am, except when I do something stupid (and I do), entirely pain free. I own a small restaurant, where I also cook. I can spend ten hours on my feet with the fryolators gurgling and the customers screaming and go home pain-free. But it is more than that. My self-image has been transformed. I no longer feel like the person who can't help move a couch. I no longer wonder whether a hike is going to cause me pain. Although people in my classes might beg to differ, I feel supple. I can bend like a reed.

I am very grateful for my YMAA training, particularly for the relaxation of my spine. It has freed me from pain and shown me a path to feeling healthy.

**Jeff Rosen**
**Tai chi instructor**

# THE
# PAIN-FREE BACK

**Westfield Memorial Library**
Westfield, New Jersey

# DR. YANG, JWING-MING

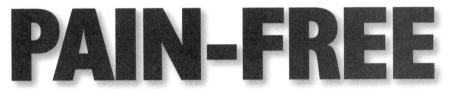

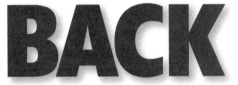

54 Simple Qigong Movements for
Healing and Prevention

YMAA Publication Center
Wolfeboro, NH USA

**YMAA Publication Center, Inc.**
PO Box 480
Wolfeboro, New Hampshire, 03894
1-800-669-8892 • info@ymaa.com • www.ymaa.com

ISBN: 9781594395376 (print) • ISBN: 9781594395383 (ebook)

Copyright ©2017 by Dr. Yang, Jwing-Ming
All rights reserved including the right of reproduction in whole or in part in any form.
Edited by Leslie Takao and Doran Hunter
Cover design by Axie Breen
Photos by the author unless noted otherwise
This book typeset in 11.5 pt Minion Pro Regular
Typesetting by Westchester Publishing Services
Illustrations provided by the author unless otherwise noted.

10  9  8  7  6  5  4  3  2  1

Printed in Canada

**Publisher's Cataloging in Publication**

Names: Yang, Jwing-Ming, 1946– author.
Title: The pain-free back : 54 easy qigong movements for healing / Dr. Yang, Jwing-Ming. —
Other titles: Back pain relief.
Description: Wolfeboro NH USA : YMAA Publication Center, Inc., [2017] | "This
  book . . . is an abridgement of the larger book by Dr. Yang, Jwing-Ming titled 'Back pain
  relief: qigong exercises for healing and prevention'. This version highlights the exercises
  you need to treat your back pain, leaving the richness of qigong healing history to the
  preceding fuller edition."—Note from the Publisher.
Identifiers: ISBN: 9781594395376 (print) | 9781594395383 (ebook) | LCCN: 2017949055
Subjects: LCSH: Backache—Exercise therapy. | Qi gong. | Backache—Alternative
  treatment. | Backache—Prevention. | BISAC: HEALTH & FITNESS / Pain Management. |
  BODY, MIND & SPIRIT / Healing / Energy (Qigong, Reiki, Polarity) | HEALTH &
  FITNESS / Diseases / Musculoskeletal. | HEALTH & FITNESS / Exercise. | SPORTS &
  RECREATION / Health & Safety.
Classification: LCC: RD771.B217 Y213 2017 | DDC: 617.5/64062—dc23

**Disclaimer:**

The practice, treatments, and methods described in this book should not be used as an
alternative to professional medical diagnosis or treatment. The author and publisher of
this book are NOT RESPONSIBLE in any manner whatsoever for any injury or negative
effects that may occur through following the instructions and advice contained herein.

It is recommended that before beginning any treatment or exercise program, you consult
your medical professional to determine whether you should undertake this course of
practice.

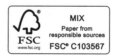

# Romanization of Chinese Words

The interior of this book primarily uses the Pinyin romanization system of Chinese to English. In some instances, a more popular word may be used as an aid for reader convenience, such as "tai chi" in place of the Pinyin spelling, *taiji*. Pinyin is standard in the People's Republic of China and in several world organizations, including the United Nations. Pinyin, which was introduced in China in the 1950s, replaces the older Wade-Giles and Yale systems.

Some common conversions are found in the following:

| Pinyin | Also spelled as | Pronunciation |
|---|---|---|
| qi | chi | chē |
| qigong | chi kung | chē gōng |
| qin na | chin na | chǐn nǎ |
| jin | jing | jǐn |
| gongfu | kung fu | gōng foo |
| taijiquan | tai chi chuan | tī jē chǔén |

For more information, please refer to *The People's Republic of China: Administrative Atlas, The Reform of the Chinese Written Language,* or a contemporary manual of style.

## Formats and Treatment of Chinese Words

The first instances of foreign words in the text proper are set in italics. Transliterations are provided frequently: for example, Eight Pieces of Brocade (Ba Duan Jin, 八段錦).

Chinese persons' names are mostly presented in their more popular English spelling. Capitalization is according to the *Chicago Manual of Style* 16th edition. The author or publisher may use a specific spelling or capitalization in respect to the living or deceased person. For example: Cheng, Man-ch'ing can be written as Zheng Manqing.

# Note from the Publisher

This book, *The Pain-Free Back*, is an abridgement of the larger book by Dr. Yang, Jwing-Ming titled *Back Pain Relief: Qigong Exercises for Healing and Prevention*. This version highlights the exercises you need to treat your back pain, the richness of qigong's healing history is available in the preceding fuller edition.

# Table of Contents

# Foreword

Ever since primitive man and woman reared up from their knuckles into the upright posture, the groan of "My aching back!" has echoed down the corridors of history in workplaces, homes, and hospitals. There are many reasons for this historical fact, a number of which have to do with lifestyle changes, fitness, and the modern environment, all of which were spelled out by Dr. Yang in the preface to his first edition and again in the preface to this revised edition. Not only does the back "carry" the body, but it also "carries" many of the psychological tensions stemming from our modern life.

In my psychiatric training, I learned this: to look at posture and body position for clues to a person's mental state—the stooped back whose owner seemed bowed by the weight of depression, the shoulders drawn in and tight and the head retracted like a turtle's in anticipation of the blow that comes only in the patient's imagination, and similar signs.

In my medical training, I learned this: back pain is one of the hardest conditions to treat effectively. The most common approaches—protracted bed rest, lying on a firm surface, time off from work—are extremely difficult for the average person to follow. Noncompliance with the regimen is extremely common. Pain medications work somewhat but risk addiction. Muscle relaxants work somewhat but have troubling side effects. Surgery works as a last resort but can make some cases worse. As a young doctor, my heart would sink whenever a case of lower back pain came into the clinical emergency room, because each one carried with it the specter of the failure of Western medicine.

In my gongfu training with Dr. Yang, I learned this: he is a dedicated scholar and a gifted teacher. He merits the highest praise, however, for his efforts to meld Eastern and Western medical understanding in hopes of achieving greater synergy between the two—in hopes that the two worldviews, combined, will be greater than the sum of their parts.

To this end, he has thoroughly revised the first edition of this book, which featured his comprehensive and wide-ranging exploration of qi theory from its historical to its present context; of the structure and function of the back; and of the Western and Eastern approaches to healing it. In addition, he has added some new concepts for explaining qi and qigong from the Western point of view. These changes further express Dr. Yang's lifelong aim of connecting Chinese and Western medical science. Finally, Dr. Yang has discovered that some of the strenuous exercises described in the first edition—which might tax persons with serious back pain—can be done from the floor instead of from a vertical stance; additional approaches for this posture have been supplied in the current revised edition.

This edition continues the approach of the previous version in that the first chapter alone serves as an excellent and clear introduction to the basic Eastern medical and martial arts idea of qi. So well-structured is this discussion that it requires no previous familiarity with this concept. The remainder of the book employs clear descriptions, relevant illustrations, and well-organized instructions to achieve the goal of providing protection and relief from back pain.

Finally, martial arts are inseparable from morality. In the present context, Dr. Yang compassionately but firmly, like a great sports coach, warns against the moral pitfalls of impatience, laziness, and fear. He encourages readers to strive to stretch their limits—carefully!—to master pain and weakness in the back. The book you hold in your hands is a noteworthy contribution to this goal.

**Thomas G. Gutheil, MD, professor of psychiatry,**
**Harvard Medical School**

# Preface

Our lifestyle continues to change from the way it was for over a million years. Now we sleep late, have less labor-intensive work, walk very little, have fewer children in our families, spend more time watching television and computer screens, and receive more radiation. Our bodies cannot adjust in a short period of time; therefore, it is difficult for us to adapt to these new, fast-developing lifestyles. Consequently, many problems occur. We have started to experience more knee pain and weakness, back degeneration and disease, breast cancer, and many other illnesses.

Today, back pain is considered by many to be one of the most serious health problems affecting quality of life. In fact, lower back pain is the second most common cause of pain, surpassed only by headaches, and is second to the common cold as a reason for doctor's office visits in the United States. It is estimated that thirty-one million Americans experience back pain at an annual cost of $16 billion to $20 billion in medical treatments and disability payments. The reason there are more back pain cases today than years ago is simply because we now use more machinery to replace our daily muscular work. Our torsos have become significantly weakened.

Therefore, if we are not aware of the problems generated by our new lifestyle and we fail to keep our torsos healthy and fit, we will most likely experience back pain before our fortieth birthdays. The key to maintaining the health of your torso is very simple: exercise correctly and stick with it. Constant exercise will slow down the aging and degeneration of the spine and build up stronger torso muscles to support the body. This is the most basic and important key to preventing back problems.

I have been studying martial qigong since I was fifteen years old. Since then, from my experience with practice and teaching, I have discovered that, among all of the qigong I have learned, the spinal qigong exercises and meditation from White Crane and taijiquan styles can heal spine problems and rebuild the strength of the torso. White Crane is considered to be a soft-hard martial style, while taijiquan is considered a soft style. In these two styles, the spine and chest are seen as two major bows, which can generate great martial power. In order to have this power, the condition of the spine and chest is extremely important. You must learn how to move them softly, like a silken whip, while coordinating the movements with your concentrated mind and breath. You must also know how to tense the torso, so that when the power reaches the target, your spine is not injured.

In these martial arts, through hundreds of years of practice and development, spine injury sometimes occurred due to the heavy training. Therefore, self-healing and conditioning of the spine have always been essential practices in White Crane and taijiquan.

Since 1986 I have conducted seminars in many countries and have taught these spinal qigong techniques for health purposes. The original purpose was to help some karate practitioners in France regain their spinal health, which they had injured through karate practice. Later, I realized these lower back problems were very common among karate practitioners due to the strenuous training. Countless people have told me how they have benefited from these simple spinal qigong exercises. I now realize that this qigong can not only heal and rebuild the spine but can also heal asthma, stomach problems, kidney irregularities, and, most important of all, strengthen the body's immune system.

I paid no attention to these qigong exercises between 1974 and 1984. During these ten years, I was busy studying for my doctorate and working as an engineer. It was not until late 1983 when I developed a kidney stone that I realized I was out of shape. When the doctor told me I would most likely experience a recurrence of the kidney stone every six months, I was very frightened because of the intense pain involved. On January 1, 1984, I quit my engineering job. I then resumed my White Crane spinal qigong practice and started to move the torso muscles above the kidneys. In Chinese qigong, to tense and relax these two muscles on the kidneys is known as a kidney massage, and through correct spinal movement, the qi and blood circulation in the kidneys can be made smooth. Amazingly, since then, I have not experienced another kidney stone.

Since the first edition of this book was published, I have received many thanks from readers and seminar participants around the world for the benefits they received from the practices introduced in it. In their conversations with me, all of these people have made the same observation: you cannot practice off and on or just for a short period of time. You must be consistent, patient, and perseverant. Usually, after three months of practice, you can feel some improvement, and after six months, you see significant improvement or complete correction of the problem.

From my additional years of teaching in seminars, I have discovered and developed a few new movements that are especially beneficial for those who already have serious back pain. I have come to realize that many people who suffer serious back pain find it difficult to do some moving exercises. Later, through pondering and teaching, I discovered that doing the same exercises while reclining on the floor can help to reestablish a healthy condition of the back. I am presenting these updated exercises and the new information I have gained.

I believe that if the Western medical community can put some effort into experimenting with ancient healing methods as a complementary medicine, conventional medical treatment will be more complete and effective. Traditional medicine originated and evolved its approach from repeated experiences over thousands of years, while modern medicines were developed from systematic study, experimentation, and research. If both approaches are useful, they should be able to cooperate with each other and complement each other.

This book is written to share my experience with those who need to heal the spine and rebuild its strength. I deeply believe that anyone, as long as he or she is patient and consistent with qigong exercises, will see positive results *within three months*. Naturally, this is not an easy task. It is a challenge to your health, happiness, and joy in life.

**Dr. Yang, Jwing-Ming**

# How to Use This Book

QIGONG IS AN ancient Chinese art of movement. These movements are simple, but their health benefits are profound. In moving the body, we also move the blood, improving both quantity and quality of qi (energy) and strengthening the muscles. This promotes mental and respiratory wellness, and your mind and breath are critical to restoring your body's energy system to a healthy state, free of blockage and pain.

My goal in writing this book is simple: to share these healing principles in a program that is straightforward and easy to use. *The Pain-Free Back* is for anyone with an ounce or more of back pain who is willing to put a little time and effort into his or her own care. If you are under forty years old and your back sometimes hurts, it is time to be proactive. If you are over forty and your back usually hurts, it is time to deal with the problem.

Maybe you have tried to deal with back pain using conventional means and you have not had good results. If so, the qigong approach is probably what you've been missing. Follow the instructions in this book. If a particular movement causes pain, do not push it. Listen to your body. Be disciplined, but also have patience.

Spine movement is the key to maintaining spinal health. It is also the key to strengthening your immune system. Make qigong a part of your life. This is the best way I know to cure back pain—and to prevent it from returning.

# Introduction

**I**T IS BELIEVED THAT the majority of adults—80 percent or more—will experience at least one significant episode of lower back pain at some point in their lives. It affects men and women alike, usually occurring between the late twenties and fifties, the middle working years. As is now known, lower back pain is the second most common cause of pain next to headaches and is second only to the common cold as a reason for office visits to primary care physicians in the United States. Once your spine is injured, it is four times more likely to get hurt again.

In order to solve this problem, we must know its causes and not just look for a cure. In our modern lifestyle, labor-intensive work has been significantly reduced and replaced by automation. Our physical body, which has evolved over millions of years to be mobile, has started to degenerate and weaken quickly.

In order to prevent further loss of our back strength, first we must study our lifestyles. No matter what, we will always be a part of nature and must follow the "natural way"—the Dao. Chinese qigong was developed by following the Dao, discerned through observation of the relationships between nature and humanity. It is a science with a solid theoretical and empirical foundation.

The most fundamental principle of Chinese medicine is the concept of qi, known today in the West as bioelectricity. Illnesses are diagnosed by evaluating the condition of the body's qi and interpreting the visible physical symptoms. According to Chinese medicine, when the need for qi and its supply in the body start to become unbalanced, the physical body is affected and can be damaged. This can happen both if the body is too yin (deficient in qi) or too yang (having an excess of qi). When practitioners of Chinese medicine diagnose any disease or condition, they explore how and where the qi is unbalanced. Once the qi imbalance is corrected and the qi returned to its normal level, the root cause of the illness has been removed. Acupuncture is a common method for adjusting the qi and preventing further physical damage. The qi level can also be raised or lowered for healing.

While Western medicine has developed according to the principle of diagnosing visible symptoms and curing visible physical damage, Chinese medicine may be more advanced in that it deals with the body's qi, the root of health. On the other hand, Chinese medicine is still far behind Western medicine in the study and research of the physical aspects of the human body. This can be seen in Western scientific methods and in the technology the West has developed. Because of the differences between the two systems of medicine, there are still large gaps in mankind's understanding of the body. I believe that if both medical cultures can learn and borrow from each other, these remaining gaps can soon be filled, and medicine as a whole will be able to take a giant step forward.

The ease of communication and the increased friendship among different cultures has given mankind an unprecedented opportunity to share such things as medical concepts. We should all take advantage of this and open our minds to the knowledge and experiences of other peoples. I sincerely hope that this takes place, especially in the field of medicine. This goal has been my motivation in writing this book. Because of my limited knowledge, I can offer only this little volume. I hope, however, that it generates widening ripples of interest in sharing and exchanging with other cultures.

In this book, we begin with the traditional Chinese approach to diagnosing and treating back pain. Next, in chapter 2, we will study the structure of our back, both physically and from Chinese qi concepts. In chapter 3, the possible causes of back pain will be discussed. Chapter 4 will review treatments by Western doctors, and chapter 5 will summarize possible treatments of back pain by practitioners of Chinese medicine. Finally, qigong exercises for back pain and rehabilitation will be introduced in chapter 6.

# CHAPTER 1

# How Do the Chinese Treat Back Pain?

## 1-1. Introduction

Qigong is the study of qi. This means that qigong actually covers a very wide field of research and includes the study of the three general types of qi (heaven qi, earth qi, and human qi) and their interrelationships. However, because the Chinese have traditionally paid more attention to the study of human qi, which is concerned with health and longevity, the term "qigong" has often been misunderstood and misused to mean only the study of human qi. Because so much attention has been given to human qi over thousands of years, human qigong has reached a very high level. Today it includes many fields such as acupuncture, herbal study, massage, cavity press, qigong exercises, martial arts, and even spiritual enlightenment.

In this chapter, I would like to summarize some of the methods commonly used in China to prevent back pain and to cure it. I would then like to focus on how qigong uses exercises and massage (including cavity press) to prevent and cure back pain.

## 1-2. Chinese Diagnosis and Treatment

Since the Western public tends to be unfamiliar with Chinese diagnosis, in this section we will first summarize the general diagnostic techniques in Chinese medicine. Then, we will review a specific diagnosis for back pain. After this, we will discuss general treatments for back pain in Chinese medicine.

## General Chinese Medical Diagnosis

When a person is sick, his qi circulation is irregular or abnormal—it has too much yin or too much yang. Because all qi channels are connected to the surface of the body, stagnant or abnormal qi flow will cause signs to show on the skin. Also, the sounds a sick person makes when speaking, coughing, or breathing are different from those of a healthy person. Chinese doctors therefore examine a patient's skin, particularly the forehead, eyes, ears, and tongue. They also pay close attention to the person's sounds. In addition, they ask the patient a number of questions about his daily habits, feeling, and activities to understand the background of the illness. Finally, the doctor feels the pulses and probes special spots on the body to further check the condition of specific channels. Therefore, Chinese diagnosis is divided into four principal categories: 1. looking (wang zhen), 2. listening and smelling (wen zhen), 3. asking (wen zhen), and 4. palpation (qie zhen).

Obviously, Chinese medicine takes a somewhat different approach to diagnosis than Western medicine. Chinese doctors treat the body as a whole, analyzing the cause of the illness from the patient's appearance and behavior. Often what the Chinese physician considers important clues or causes are viewed by the Western doctor as symptomatic or irrelevant, and vice versa.

Next, we will briefly discuss the above four Chinese diagnostic techniques.

## Looking (Wang Zhen)

Looking at the spirit and inspecting the color.

1. General appearance: Examine the facial expression, muscle tone, posture, and general spirit.

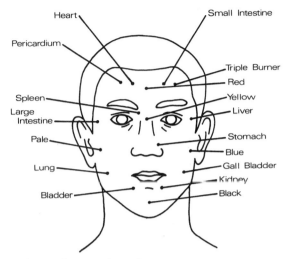

■ Diagnosis from the Face's Color

2. Skin color: Examine the skin color of the injured area, if the problem is externally visible, like a bruise or pulled muscle. Examine the skin color of the face. Because some channels are connected to the face, its color can tell the Chinese doctor what organs are disordered or out of balance.

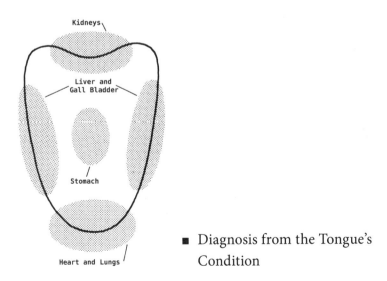

■ Diagnosis from the Tongue's Condition

3. Tongue: The tongue is closely connected through channels with the heart, kidney, stomach, liver, gall bladder, lungs, and spleen. In making his diagnosis, the Chinese doctor will check the shape, fur, color, and the body of the tongue to determine the condition of the organs.

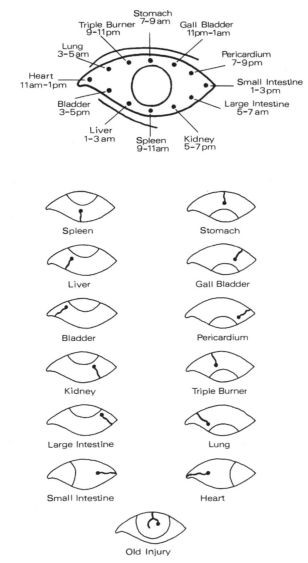

■ Diagnosis from the Eye's Black (or Blue) Spots and Lines

4. Eyes: From the appearance of the eyes a doctor can tell the liver condition. For example, when the eyes are red, it means the liver has too much yang. Also, black spots on the whites of the eyes can tell of problems with the qi circulation, degeneration of organs, or stagnancy due to an old injury.

5. Hair: The condition of the hair can indicate the health of the kidneys and the blood. For example, thin, dry hair indicates deficient kidney qi or weak blood.

6. Lip and gums: The color of the lips and their relative dryness indicate if the qi is deficient or exhausted. Red, swollen, or bleeding gums can be caused by stomach fire. Pale, swollen gums and loose teeth might be a symptom of deficient kidneys.

# Listening and Smelling (Wen Zhen)

1. Listening to a patient's breathing, mode of speech, and cough. For example, a dry, hacking cough is caused by dry heat in the lungs.

2. Smelling the odor of a patient's breath and excrement. For example, in the case of diseases caused by excessive heat, the various secretions and excretions of the body have a heavy, foul odor, while in diseases caused by excessive cold, they smell more like rotten fish.

# Asking (Wen Zhen)

This is one of the most important sources of a successful diagnosis. The questions usually cover the patient's past medical history, present condition, habits, and lifestyle. Traditionally, there are ten main subjects a Chinese doctor will focus on in this interview. They are as follows:

1. Chills and fever
2. Head and body

3. Perspiration

4. Diet and appetite

5. Urine and stool

6. Chest and abdomen

7. Eyes and ears

8. Sleep

9. Medical history

10. Bearing and living habits

# Palpation (Qie Zhen)

There are three major forms of palpation (touching or feeling) in Chinese medicine:

1. The palpation of areas that feel painful, hot, or swollen to determine the nature of the problem. For example, swelling and heat indicate that there is too much yang in the area.

2. The palpation of specific acupuncture points on the front and back of the trunk. For example, if an area feels collapsed or the point is sore to the touch, there could be disease in the organ with which the point is associated.

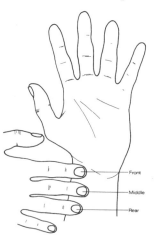

Front
Middle
Rear

■ The Palpation of the Pulse

3. The palpation of the pulse. Traditionally, the radial pulse on the wrist is the principal site for pulse diagnosis. Although the pulse is specially related to the lungs and controlled by the heart, it signals the condition of all organs. The doctor checks the following: the depth (floating or submerged), the pace (slow or fast), the length (long or short), the strength (weak or strong), and the quality (slippery, rough, wiry, tight, huge, fine, or irregular). Usually, it takes several years and hundreds of cases to become expert in the palpation of the pulse.

| The Palpation of the Pulse | |
|---|---|
| **Left Hand** | **Organs** |
| Rear | Kidney Yin |
| Middle | Liver |
| Front | Heart |
| **Right Hand** | **Organs** |
| Rear | Kidney Yang |
| Middle | Spleen |
| Front | Lungs |

Recently, inspection of skin eruptions on the ears has been used in Chinese diagnosis. A number of sites have been found on the ear that become spontaneously tender or otherwise react to disease or injury somewhere in the body. Stimulation of these ear points in turn exerts certain therapeutic effects on those parts of the body with which they are associated. Moreover, many Western diagnostic methods, such as using X-rays, have also been adopted to coordinate with Chinese diagnosis.

This section serves as only a brief introduction to Chinese medical diagnosis. Interested readers should refer to books about Chinese medicine for more information.

Next, we will list the possible diagnostic techniques for back pain. However, before we begin, first let us see how the Chinese define back pain or pain associated with the back. The most common term for back pain is yaotong (lumbago)—waist pain. From this, you can see most back pain is in the waist area (i.e., lumbar vertebrae). It is also called yaokaotong (lumbosacral pain)—pain in the lumbar vertebrae. However, when the pain has reached to the upper section of the spine, it is called yaojitong—pain along the spinal column. If the pain in the waist area is only sore without severe pain, it is called yaosuan—soreness of waist. And if the entire back is aching, it is called yaobeitengtong—pain in the back and loins, lumbago and back pain.

From this terminology, you can see that according to Chinese medical definitions, back pain is not a disease, but the pain is caused by some special sickness. Therefore, the beginning treatment is to stop the pain and then follow with some herbal treatments or special qigong exercises to heal the sickness or to rebuild the strength of the physical and qi bodies. It is believed that only then will the root of the sickness be removed and further sickness prevented.

# Diagnosis for Back Pain

1. Looking and inspecting the posture of the patient to see if there is any abnormal structure in or appearance of the spine.

2. Asking the patient about, and understanding, the patient's medical history and conditions. Where is the pain? How did the back pain start? How long have the symptoms existed? When is the pain most serious?

3. Palpating the areas that feel painful, hot, and swollen, to determine the nature of the problem. Also, from the hands' touch on special areas or cavities on the back, an experienced Chinese physician is able to tell where the qi is stagnant on the back.

4. From different angles of arm or leg movement or different angles of the torso's gentle twisting and bending, identifying some special injuries or muscular spasms.

## General Chinese Treatments for Back Pain

As mentioned earlier, back pain is not considered to be a sickness but a pain caused by other sicknesses. Therefore, the usual treatment is first to stop the pain by using acupuncture, massage, or both in combination. The key to reaching this goal is to improve the qi and blood circulation in the pained area. Occasionally, herbs are also used to improve the circulation and stop the pain. However, all of these measures are considered temporary, because they are not able to cure the root of the sickness but only alleviate the symptoms. In order to have a complete recovery or cure the root of the problem, a healthy and strong foundation must be rebuilt. Naturally, this usually takes a long time, but it is a long-term solution.

Therefore, on the one hand, a Chinese physician will treat the painful symptoms and try to make the patient more comfortable, while on the other hand he will teach the patient some special qigong breathing techniques and movements to either expedite the recovery from sickness or to rebuild the strength of the body.

As a matter of fact, the best way to maintain health is to prevent sickness from occurring. It is the same for back pain. The best way to prevent it from occurring is to be aware of your lifestyle and to keep your body in good condition. However, if it has already occurred, then the appropriate course is to prevent it from getting any worse and learn to rebuild the physical strength of the back so that it can resume functioning normally.

The Chinese developed numerous methods for treating back pain. In this section, we will briefly discuss the theory behind those. In chapter 6, we will learn numerous qigong exercises for treating back pain.

**Massage.** When done properly, massage will improve the qi and blood circulation in the joint areas. Once this circulation is improved, the pain can be eased and the patient able to feel more comfortable.

Generally speaking, Chinese massage can be classified into four categories according to their purposes. They are as follows:

1. **General Massage (Pu Tong An Mo).** General massage is the most common and popular massage. The purposes of general massage are simple, and the techniques are relatively easier than the other three categories. The six main goals of this massage are relaxation, recovery from fatigue, preventing illness, slowing down aging, speeding recovery from sudden environmental qi disturbance, and enjoyment.

From these, you can see that general massage is not aiming for healing but for improving the qi and blood circulation for different purposes. Normally, a Chinese massage therapist will start his or her training from general massage. This is simply because through general massage practice, you can master the basic massage techniques and also get a better acquaintance with the human anatomy and the qi status of the body. If you wish to know more about Chinese massage, please refer to the book *Chinese Qigong Massage: General Massage*, published by YMAA.

2. **Push Grab Massage (Tui Na An Mo).** Tui na massage is often simply called tui na. Tui na means "push" and "grab" and refers to the two major techniques. Tui na has two main purposes: treating injuries and treating illnesses, especially in small children. When tui na is used for treating injuries, the main goal is to remove any blood stagnation (i.e., bruises) and qi blockage, thereby expediting the healing process. When it is used for treating sickness, the main goal is to regulate the abnormal qi circulation of the internal organs to a healthy state.

3.  **Cavity Press Massage (Dian Xue An Mo).** Cavity press (dian xue) is the method of using the fingertips (especially the thumb tip) to press acupuncture cavities and certain other points (pressure points) on the body in order to manipulate the qi circulation. Acupuncture cavities are tiny spots distributed over the entire body where the qi of the body can be manipulated through massage or the insertion of needles. According to the new theory of bioelectricity, these cavities are places where the electrical conductivity is higher than in neighboring areas. They are therefore more sensitive to external stimulation and allow it to reach to the primary qi channels.

The theory of cavity press is very similar to that of acupuncture. There are a few differences, however. Acupuncture uses needles or other means of penetration such as lasers, while cavity press uses the fingertips to press the cavities. Acupuncture can reach much deeper than cavity press. Cavity press, though, is easier and more convenient than acupuncture, which requires equipment and a higher level of training. This means that anyone can learn to use cavity press to treat back pain after only a short period of training and some experience, while acupuncture takes years of study to learn. A patient can use cavity press on himself or herself much more easily than acupuncture.

In cavity press, stagnant qi deep in the joint can be led to the surface. This improves the qi circulation in the joint area and reduces pain considerably. The use of cavity press to speed up the healing of injured joints is very common in the Chinese martial arts.

4.  **Qi Massage (Qi An Mo).** Qi massage is commonly called wai qi liao fa, which means "curing with external qi," and is commonly translated as "qi healing" in the West today. This term implies that the massage is done through qi correspondence rather than touch.

To understand qi massage, you must recognize that qi is the bio-electricity circulating in the body. Because it is electricity, it can be conducted or led through electrical correspondence. Actually, everybody has the ability to do qi healing. For example, when your friend is sad, his qi status is yin (i.e., deficient). If you hold his hands or hug him, your qi will nourish him, and he will immediately feel better. Humans have been doing this instinctively for a long time. The only difference between the average person and a qigong master is that the latter has trained in qi healing and can therefore be more effective.

In qi massage, a patient's back pain can be alleviated when the accumulated or stagnant qi is led away from the painful area. This will make the patient more relaxed and feel more comfortable. Naturally, like other massage, the healing process can be expedited. If you are interested in knowing more about Chinese massage, please refer to the book *Chinese Qigong Massage: General Massage*, published by YMAA.

**Acupuncture.** Acupuncture is another common method of temporarily stopping the pain and increasing the qi circulation in the joint area to help the healing. The main difference between massage and acupuncture is that the former usually stays only on the surface, while the latter can reach to the center of the joint. One of the advantages of acupuncture is that if the back pain is caused by an old injury deep in the joint, it can heal the injury or at least remove some of the stagnated qi or bruising.

In acupuncture, needles or other newly developed means such as lasers or electricity are used to stimulate and increase the qi circulation. Although acupuncture can stop the pain and can, to some degree, cure back pain, the process can be so time-consuming as to be emotionally draining. Acupuncture is an external method, and while it may remove the symptoms, it can usually heal back pain only temporarily or only to a limited degree. Rebuilding the strength of the joints in the spine is a long-term proposition. Therefore, after back pain patients have received some treatment, the physician will frequently encourage them to get involved in qigong exercises to rebuild the joints.

**Herbal Treatments.** Herbal treatments are used together with massage and acupuncture, especially when back pain is caused by an injury. The herbs are usually made into a plaster or ground into powder, mixed with a liquid such as alcohol, and then applied to the joint. The dressing is changed every twenty-four hours.

Herbal treatments are used to alleviate pain, to increase the qi circulation and help the healing of injury, and to speed up the process of regrowth. Often, oral herbs are prescribed by a Chinese physician to stop the pain and also to expedite the healing process.

**Qigong Exercises.** The main purpose of qigong exercise for back pain is to rebuild the strength of the joint by improving the qi circulation. As mentioned earlier, traditional Chinese physicians believe that because the body's cells are alive, as long as there is a proper supply of qi, physical damage can be repaired or even completely rebuilt. They have proven that broken bones can be mended completely, even in the elderly. Even some Western physicians have now come to believe that damaged or degenerated joints can be regrown back to their original healthy state.[2]

Let us now summarize the similarities and differences in how Chinese and Western medicines treat back pain.

# Summary

## Diagnosis

1. Neither Western nor Chinese diagnosis can pinpoint the cause of back pain clearly.

2. Western diagnosis is more detailed, and disease or injury is diagnosed using the theory that seeing is believing. Therefore, all diagnoses originate from an anatomical point of view.

Different high-tech instruments have been developed and used to see internal physical problems. However, although Chinese medicine today also uses X-rays for diagnosis, traditionally the diagnosis depended on surface appearance and feeling.

3. In Western diagnosis, different terminology has been created to explain the possible causes of back pain. There are not many different terms in Chinese medicine for back pain. In Chinese medicine, normally the causes of back pain are identified as only muscle or tendon spasm, qi stagnation, bone's fracture, ligament's injury, arthritis, or a combination of these factors. From this, you can see that it is much clearer to identify different causes of back pain from a Western point of view.

## Treatments

1. Both Western and Chinese medicine use massage to alleviate pain by improving qi and blood circulation.

2. Western medicine uses both ice and heat to ease pain and inflammation, while Chinese medicine uses only heat. This is because Chinese doctors believe that the ice treatment can only slow down the qi and blood circulation and make the qi and blood condense deeper into the joint, thus hindering the healing process.

3. Western medicine uses drugs to make the body relax and to ease pain. However, side effects have been widely noticed. Chinese medicine often uses acupuncture and external herbal treatments to ease pain, keep swelling down, and to improve qi and blood circulation. Occasionally, internal herbs are used to reduce swelling, remove bruises, prevent further infection of the joints, and to expedite healing by improving qi and blood circulation. Normally, there are no or very minimal side effects from Chinese herbal treatments.

4. Western medicine teaches patients physical exercises to strengthen and rebuild the spine. However, Chinese qigong teaches patients how to use the mind, coordinated with breathing techniques, to enhance the qi storage and circulation internally while also using physical qigong movements to rebuild the strength and health of the vertebrae. A more detailed discussion of the differences between using Western physical exercise and Chinese qigong for spinal rejuvenation will appear in the next section.

5. Western medicine is not concerned with qi status when a patient has a back pain problem. However, Chinese medicine pays great attention to it. Teaching a patient how to rebuild the qi level and enhance the qi circulation in the injured area has been considered an important key to the healing process.

## Prevention

In Western medicine and health care, little has been written about how to prevent back pain from occurring. It was not until the last two decades that there was much information available on the possible factors responsible for causing such pain and how to prevent it.

However, strengthening the torso has always been an important part of qigong practice in China. From past experience, it is understood that if the physical torso is not strong and the qi circulation is not abundant in the center, the immune system will be weak and a person can sicken easily. On the one hand, qigong teaches a practitioner how to build up the qi and, with the coordination of the breathing, use the mind to enhance its circulation. On the other hand, it emphasizes the health of the physical body.

In the next section, we will discuss in more detail how qigong massage and exercise can prevent and cure back pain. We will also summarize the differences between the Western and Chinese qigong approaches.

# 1-3. How Can Qigong Cure Back Pain?

Due to a lack of knowledge and experience in acupuncture and herbal treatments in general, I will not include these two fields in our discussion. If you are interested in knowing more about the treatments from these two fields, you should refer to other related books and resources. In this section, the discussion will be limited to qigong exercise and massage.

In Chinese medicine, the concept of qi is used both in diagnosis and treatment. A basic principle of Chinese medicine is that you have to rebalance the qi before you can cure the root of a disease. Only then can you also repair the physical damage and rebuild your physical strength and health. This theory is very simple. Your entire body is made up of living cells. When these cells receive the proper qi supply, they will function normally and even repair themselves. However, if the qi supply is abnormal and this condition persists, then even though the cells were originally healthy, they will become damaged or changed (perhaps even becoming cancerous). In light of this basic qi theory, let us first discuss why qigong can be effective in curing back pain.

## Why Is Qigong Effective for Back Pain?

**Qigong Maintains and Increases Smooth Qi Circulation.** As mentioned earlier, the goal of qigong healing is to reestablish a strong, smooth flow of qi through the affected area. When this happens, physical damage can be repaired and strength rebuilt. Traditional Chinese physicians have always believed that as long as you are alive, physical damage to the body can be repaired through improving the qi and blood circulation. Most Western physicians don't agree with this and believe some conditions—for example, osteoarthritis caused by aging and the degeneration of the joints—cannot be reversed.

However, some Western physicians are beginning to change their minds about this.[2]

**Qigong Strengthens the Physical and Mental Bodies.** The greatest benefit of Chinese qigong is probably in the physical (yang) and mental (yin) training. Qigong teaches you how to regulate the mind to a calm, profound, and concentrated meditative state. It also teaches you how to use your regulated mind in coordination with deep breathing to lead the qi circulating in your body. From this internal guidance and coordination with specific qigong movements, you can either heal yourself or rebuild the strength of your physical body. From the yin (mental body) and yang (physical body) balance, you regain your health.

**Qigong Strengthens the Immune and Hormone Production Systems.** Western science knows that the body's immune system is closely related to the endocrine glands, which produce hormones. Hormones cause fundamental processes such as growth, reproduction, and sexual response to speed up or slow down. (The word "hormone" comes from a Greek word that means "to excite, to stimulate, or to stir up.") They also strengthen the ability of the immune system to fight diseases. For example, it is believed that the thymus gland (which is located just behind the top of the sternum) plays an important role in the body's immune system, but we do not have a full understanding of the function of the thymus.[3] We also still do not know very much about the pineal gland in the upper back part of the brain. In fact, it has only recently come to be believed that hormone production is significantly related to the aging process.

Many of us know of people who were deathly sick, but who had a very high spirit and a strong desire to survive, and miraculously recovered. Both Western and Eastern communities tell of many such cases. Chinese qigong practitioners believe that if a sick person can lead qi to the brain through concentration or through strong desire, he or she can evoke a powerful healing force. A possible explanation is that the stronger qi flow activates the pineal and pituitary glands so that they generate more hormones. We do know that the most important function of the pituitary gland is to stimulate, regulate, and coordinate the functions of the other endocrine glands.[3] For this reason, it is sometimes called the "master gland."

In Chinese qigong, the upper dan tian (which some Westerners refer to as the "third eye") is considered the center of your whole being. If you raise your spirit, which resides there, you can energize your body, manifest amazing physical and mental strength, and recover more quickly from injury or sickness. Certain groups in the West have also recognized its importance as the center of the spirit and consider it a "third eye," which is able to sense further than the physical eyes.

If we combine the understanding of old and new, and of East and West, we can conclude that what actually happens, probably because of mental concentration, is that a stronger current of bioelectricity is led to the pineal and pituitary glands to activate the production of hormones. This stimulates the entire endocrine system and causes it to function more effectively, improving healing, cellular regeneration, reproduction, and growth. If this is correct, then it is possible to begin a new era of scientific self-healing or spiritual healing. An alternative result is that we may learn how to devise electrical equipment to activate the pineal and pituitary glands to improve the effectiveness and speed of healing. Perhaps we may also be able to find the secret key to slowing down the aging process.

**Qigong Raises the Spirit of Vitality.** The spirit is closely tied to the mind and cannot be separated from it. In qigong practice, the mind is considered the general in the battle against sickness. When the mind (general) has a strong will, thoroughly understands the battlefield (the body), wisely and carefully sets up the strategy (the breathing technique), and effectively and efficiently manages the soldiers (the qi), then the morale (spirit) of the general and soldiers will be high. When this happens, sickness can be conquered and health regained. The best way to prevent back pain from returning once you have cured it is to make qigong part of your life.

When you use qigong to treat your back pain, you must first treat your mind by changing the way you look at your sickness and your life. Do not passively accept the negative things that have happened to you. Become more active and take charge of your life. Most basically, learn how to keep the back pain from disturbing your peace of mind. Remember, doing something is better than doing nothing.

Second, you must rebuild your confidence in your ability to treat your back pain. Even though you may have failed before, don't let that discourage you. Learn about the causes of your problem, understand the theory of this new treatment, and try to think about how you can make the treatment more effective. Once you do this, you will have rebuilt your confidence not only in the treatment but also in your life.

Third, after you have practiced qigong for a while, you will understand your body better, and you will deal with such problems more easily. You may realize that the pain is not necessarily all bad. Pain draws your attention to your body and helps you to understand yourself better. Pain can also help you to build up willpower and perseverance. However, you must first know what pain is, for only then will you stop it. This is called regulating your mind. Remember that medicine is only a temporary solution.

Once you begin to take action, build your confidence, and learn to understand your pain, you will be on your way to developing the willpower, patience, and perseverance needed to keep up with the treatment. You can see that Chinese qigong heals by going to the root of the problem. It improves the entire body, both mentally and physically, and strengthens the immune system. Only when this is done will the illness be healed completely.

# How Chinese Qigong Exercises Differ from Western Exercises

1. From a theoretical point of view, qigong originated from the concept of regulating the qi (from an imbalanced condition to a balanced one) both before and after physical damage has occurred. Western medicine, however, does not yet fully accept the existence of qi or bioelectricity and is therefore not concerned with it.

2. Chinese qigong considers the regulation of the body to be the most basic and important factor in successful practice. Regulating the body means bringing your body into a very relaxed, centered, and balanced state. Only then can your mind be calm and comfortable. When the body is relaxed, the qi can circulate freely and be led easily anywhere you wish, such as to the skin or even deep into the bone marrow and the internal organs. To cure back pain, you have to be so relaxed that you can lead the qi deep into the joint where the qi can repair the damage. Western back pain exercises are not usually specifically concerned with relaxation.

The first priority in qigong exercise for back pain is learning how to relax and avoid muscle and tendon tension and stress in the joint area, which is especially critical in cases of severe back pain. Practitioners of Chinese medicine reason that exercises that tense the muscles and tendons will inhibit the qi circulation from going deep into the damaged joint. Furthermore, tension of the muscles and tendons increases pressure on the joint and can increase the damage. Therefore, traditional Chinese physicians recommend relaxed, gentle movements as a first step to smoothly increase the qi circulation. Only when the patient has rebuilt the strength of the joint will the muscles and tendons be exercised. After all, strong muscles and tendons are what will prevent future joint damage.

However, in Western physical exercise for back pain, before any healing or rehabilitation of the deep joint area is done, strenuous muscle and tendon strengthening exercises have already been conducted. From a Chinese qigong point of view, knowing the correct way of exercising from soft to hard is a key to rebuilding the healthy condition of the joints from deep within to the surface.

3. With qigong, in addition to the body being relaxed, the breathing must be long, deep, and calm. As we noted above, according to qigong theory, breathing is the strategy of your practice. When you exhale, you instinctively and naturally lead qi to the surface of your body, and when you inhale, you lead it inward to the bone marrow and the internal organs. In qigong you have to learn to breathe deeply and calmly in coordination with your thinking. This way, your mind can lead the qi strongly into the damaged area. In Western exercise for back pain, coordinating the deep breathing with the movement is not emphasized.

4. Because the mind is one of the major forces of qi or bioelectric circulation—mind is in fact an electromotive force—it has an important role in healing. In order to make your qigong practice really effective, in addition to regulating your body and breathing, you must also regulate your mind. Regulating your mind means to lead it away from outside distractions and turn it toward feeling what is going on inside your body. In order to lead qi to the damaged places in your body, your mind must be calm, relaxed, and concentrated, so that you can feel or sense the qi. The mind, therefore, plays a very important role in qigong. Western back pain exercise, on the other hand, is usually not concerned at all with the training of the meditative mind.

5. Another significant difference between qigong and Western back pain exercise is that qigong emphasizes not only healing

the joints but also rebuilding the health of the internal organs. Remember, only when the internal organs are healthy can the root of the qi imbalance be removed and, therefore, the cause of the sickness be corrected. But qigong is not just concerned with bringing the organs back to health; it also works to strengthen them. Western back pain exercises, in contrast, are not at all concerned with the health of the internal organs.

6. One of the most significant results of qigong practice is maintaining hormone production at a healthy level, which keeps the immune system functioning effectively. In Western medicine, imbalanced hormone production is adjusted with drugs.

7. The most significant difference between qigong and Western back pain exercise is probably that practicing qigong draws the patient gradually into an acquaintance with the inner energy side of his or her body. In other words, internal self-awareness will be increased. Once this is experienced, patients can start to feel energy imbalances when they are just beginning and, consequently, can correct them before physical damage occurs. In fact, this is the key to preventing most illnesses.

You can see that although many of the movements of qigong and Western back pain exercises are similar, the theory of qigong is more profound, and therefore the challenge is more significant. In fact, the best way to maintain your health and rebuild your qi and body is by understanding the theory of qigong and starting the training. If you are interested in knowing more about qigong training, please refer to the book *The Root of Chinese Qigong*, published by YMAA.

Because this book will also introduce qigong massage for back pain, we would like to point out some of the major differences between qigong massage and regular Western massage.

# How Chinese Qigong Massage Differs from Western Massage

1. Chinese massage pays attention to improving the circulation of both qi and blood, while Western massage normally emphasizes only good blood circulation and a comfortable, easy feeling.

2. In Chinese massage, the massage therapist and the patient must communicate with each other both through touch and through deeper levels of contact. This mutual cooperation enables the massager to use his or her mind to either lead qi into the patient or to remove excess qi from the patient's body. Therefore, qigong massage requires a higher level of experience and training in concentration. This means that the massage is not limited to only a physical massage; it is also a qi massage. The most important part of this cooperation is that the patient can use his or her own mind to relax the area being massaged and make the massage more effective. Furthermore, this cooperation helps the patient to calm the mind and relax deeply into the internal organs and bone marrow, which makes it possible for the massage to regulate the qi. In Western massage, coordination between the massager and the patient is not emphasized.

3. Cavity press or acupressure techniques are considered part of qigong massage. Like Japanese shiatsu massage, which is derived from Chinese acupressure, finger pressure on the cavities is used to regulate the qi circulation and to remove qi and blood stagnation in the affected areas. To do this kind of massage effectively requires not only that the massage therapist know the location of the cavities but also that he or she also understand the twelve qi channels, how to use them to remove excess qi from affected areas, and how to bring in nourishing qi. It is also extremely helpful if the massage

therapist is experienced in qigong. This kind of practice is almost completely ignored in Western massage.

# References

1. Robert O. Becker and Gary Selden, *The Body Electric* (New York: William Morrow, 1985).
2. W. Gifford-Jones, "Keeping the Human Body Active Reduces Risk of Osteoarthritis," *Globe and Mail*, January 31, 1989.
3. Benjamin F. Miller, *The Complete Medical Guide* (New York: Simon & Schuster, 1978).

# CHAPTER 2

# Understanding Our Back

## 2-1. Introduction

In order to maintain the health of our back, or solve back pain problems, it is important to study the anatomical structure of our back, especially the spine. From this study, we can better understand the problem and its possible causes. In addition, according to Chinese medical science, many back pain problems may also be caused by qi imbalance or stagnation in the spine or back muscles. Therefore, if we are wise, we will examine our back from both a Western physical understanding and also from the Eastern notion of qi distribution in our back.

## 2-2. The Qi Network in Our Back

We have two bodies, the physical body and the qi body (or bioelectric body). The physical body can be seen, but qi can only be felt. The qi body is the vital source of the physical body (i.e., any alive cells) and the foundation of our lives. The qi body is not only related to our cells but also to our thinking and spirit, because it is the main energy source for maintaining the brain's functioning. Therefore, any qi imbalance or stagnation will be the root and cause of any physical sickness or mental disorder.

Western medical science has long been studying the physical body and ignoring the qi body for the most part. Although this has begun to change in recent decades, the scientific understanding of the qi body and how it affects our health and longevity is still in its infancy. Under these circumstances, we may still accept the ancient Chinese understanding of our body's qi network.

In this section, we will first briefly describe this network. Then, we will focus on the central energy system and central energy lines discovered through Chinese qigong and its possible linkage to newer scientific discoveries.

# Twelve Primary Qi Channels and the Eight Vessels

From the understanding of Chinese medicine, the qi circulatory system in a human body includes eight vessels (ba mai), twelve primary qi channels (shi er jing), and thousands of secondary channels branching out from the primary channels (luo). On two of the vessels (governing and conception vessels) and the twelve primary qi channels, there are more than seven hundred acupuncture cavities through which the qi level in the channels can be adjusted and regulated. From this qi adjustment, the qi circulation in the body, especially in the internal organs, can be regulated into a harmonious state, the body's sickness can be cured, and health can be maintained. Here, we will briefly review these three circulatory networks. If you are interested in learning more about this qi network, you may refer to Chinese acupuncture books or my book *The Root of Chinese Qigong*, published by YMAA.

## Eight Vessels (Ba Mai)

1. The eight vessels include four yang vessels and four yin vessels that balance each other.

2. The four yang vessels are as follows:

   - Governing Vessel (Du Mai)

   - Belt (or Girdle) Vessel (Dai Mai)

   - Heel Vessel (Yangchiao Mai)

   - Linking Vessel (Yangwei Mai)

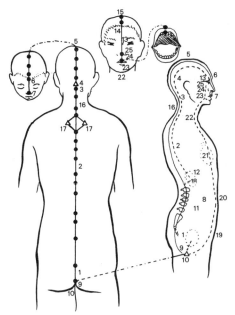

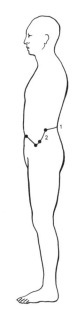

■ The Governing Vessel (Du Mai)

■ The Belt (Girdle) Vessel
(Ren Mai)

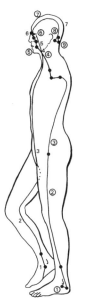

■ The Yang Heel Vessel
(Yangchiao Mai)

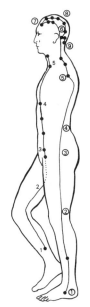

■ The Yang Linking
Vessel (Yangwei Mai)

3. The four yin vessels are as follows:

- Conception Vessel (Ren Mai)
- Thrusting Vessel (Chong Mai)
- Heel Vessel (Yinchiao Mai)
- Linking Vessel (Yinwei Mai)

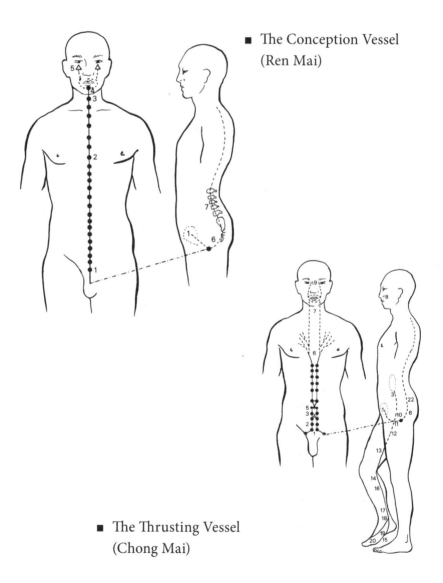

- The Conception Vessel
  (Ren Mai)

- The Thrusting Vessel
  (Chong Mai)

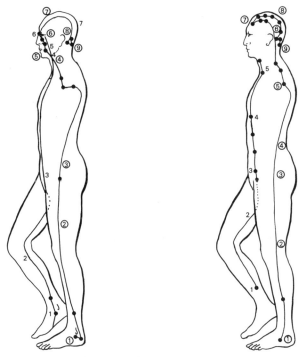

■ Heel Vessel (Yinchiao Mai)    ■ Linking Vessel (Yinwei Mai)

4. According to Chinese medicine, vessels function as reservoirs, connected to the twelve primary qi channels and regulating the qi level circulating in these channels. When the qi level in some specific channel is too high, one or more of the reservoirs will absorb the excess qi, and if the qi is too low, the shortfall will be supplied from these vessels. Consequently, a harmonious level can be maintained.

5. The two yang vessels, governing and belt vessels, and the two yin vessels, conception and thrusting vessels, are individual and are located in the torso. The other four vessels exist in pairs and are located in the legs. There are no vessels in the arms.

6. Among the eight vessels, according to Chinese medicine, the governing and conception vessels are the most important

because they are the main vessels that regulate the twelve primary qi channels. The governing vessel regulates the qi in the six primary yang qi channels, while the conception vessel regulates the qi in the six primary yin qi channels. There are acupuncture cavities on these two vessels, and none on the other six vessels. However, there are many cavities on these six vessels that belong to the twelve primary qi channels. These cavities are considered to be gates that allow the qi to pass between the vessels and channels.

7. According to Chinese qigong practice for health and longevity, learning how to fill out the qi in the vessels is very important. The reason for this is that these eight vessels are the reservoirs for the qi. When the qi in these reservoirs is abundant, the qi-regulating potential of the primary qi channels will be high and efficient. The qi circulates in the governing and conception vessels and distributes to the twelve primary qi channels (i.e., limbs) throughout the day.

8. In religious qigong meditation practice for enlightenment, the thrusting vessel (i.e., spinal cord) is very important. The thrusting vessel connects the brain and the perineum, and the qi is abundant in this vessel at around midnight. Traditionally, during the midnight hours, we are sleeping and the physical body is extremely relaxed. In this situation, the physical body does not need a great amount of qi to support its activities, and the qi circulates abundantly in the spinal cord to nourish the brain and sexual organs. Hormone production is therefore increased at night. When the brain is nourished and its function is raised to a high level, the spirit can be raised and enlightenment can be achieved. If you are interested in learning more about this subject, please refer to the book *Qigong: The Secret of Youth*, published by YMAA.

9. The governing vessel, which is located at the center of the back, is the main vessel supplying qi to the nervous system branching out from the spinal cord. The nervous system is constructed of physical cells that need to be nourished with qi (bioelectricity) to function and stay alive. This tells us that qi is ultimately the root of the nerves' functioning. To maintain abundant qi circulation in this vessel, your physical health condition is extremely important. If there is any physical injury or damage along the course of this vessel, the qi supply to the nervous system will be stagnant and irregular. Moreover, in order to have healthy and abundant qi circulation in this vessel, you must learn how to increase the storage of the qi in the lower dan tian, which is the main qi reservoir or bioelectric battery in our body.

10. The yang belt vessel is the only vessel in which the qi circulates horizontally. To qigong practitioners, this vessel is very important. Because the qi status in this vessel is yang, the qi is expanding outward. It is from this vessel that we feel our balance. It is just like an airplane or a tightrope walker: the longer the wings or the balancing pole, the easier it will be to find and maintain balance. A qigong practitioner or a Chinese martial artist will train this vessel and make the qi expand outward further, therefore increasing the balance and stability of both the physical and mental bodies. When you have more balance and stability, you can find your center. When you find your physical and mental center, then you will be rooted. Once you are rooted, your spirit can be raised to a higher level.

# The Twelve Primary Qi Channels and Their Branches (Shi Er Jing Luo)

1. The twelve primary qi channels include six yang channels and six yin channels. They balance each other.

2. The six yang channels are as follows:

- Hand Yang Brightness Large Intestine Channel (Shou Yang Ming Da Chang Jing)
- Foot Yang Brightness Stomach Channel (Zu Yang Ming Wei Jing)
- Hand Greater Yang Small Intestine Channel (Shou Tai Yang Xiao Chang Jing)
- Foot Greater Yang Bladder Channel (Zu Tai Yang Pang Guang Jing)
- Hand Lesser Yang Triple Burner Channel (Shou Shao Yang San Jiao Jing)
- Foot Lesser Yang Gall Bladder Channel (Zu Shao Yang Dan Jing)

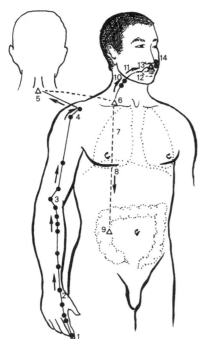 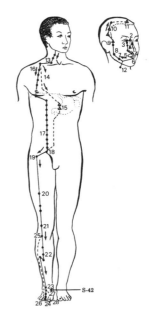

- The Large Intestine Channel of the Hand—Yang Brightness

- The Stomach Channel of the Foot—Yang Brightness (Zu Yang Ming Wei Jing)

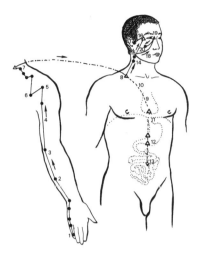

- The Small Intestine Channel of the Hand—Greater Yang (Shou Tai Yang Xiao Chang Jing)

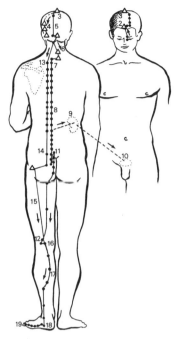

- The Urinary Bladder Channel of the Foot— Greater Yang (Zu Tai Yang Pang Guang Jing)

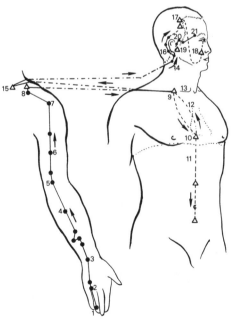

- The Triple Burner Channel of the Hand—Lesser Yang (Shou Shao Yang San Jiao Jing)

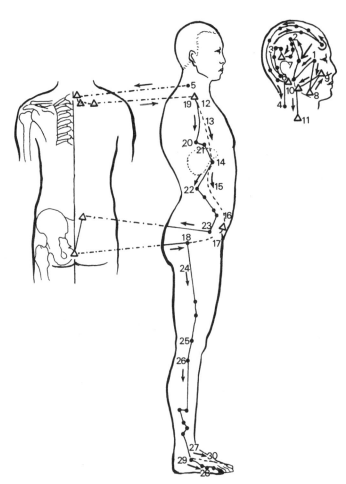

- The Gall Bladder Channel of the Foot—Lesser Yang (Zu Shao Yang Dan Jing)

3. The six yin channels are as follows:

- Hand Greater Yin Lung Channel (Shou Tai Yin Fei Jing)
- Foot Greater Yin Spleen Channel (Zu Tai Yin Pi Jing)
- Hand Lesser Yin Heart Channel (Shou Shao Yin Xin Jing)
- Foot Lesser Yin Kidney Channel (Zu Shao Yin Shen Jing)

- Hand Absolute Yin Pericardium Channel (Shou Jue Yin Xin Bao Luo Jing)

- Foot Absolute Yin Liver Channel (Zu Jue Yin Gan Jing)

4. From the illustrations above, you can see that one end of each channel connects to an extremity, and the other end connects to a different internal organ. In each channel, there are many acupuncture cavities through which the qi condition in each channel can be regulated. This is the basic theory of acupuncture.

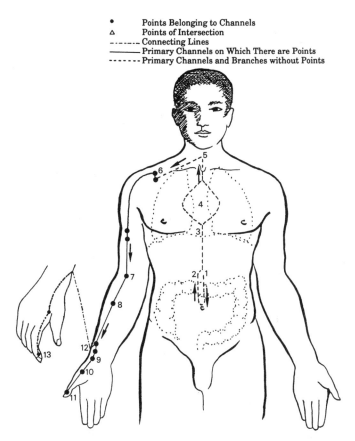

- ●   Points Belonging to Channels
- △   Points of Intersection
- ------ Connecting Lines
- ——— Primary Channels on Which There are Points
- ------ Primary Channels and Branches without Points

- The Lung Channel of the Hand—Greater Yin (Shou Tai Yin Fei Jing)

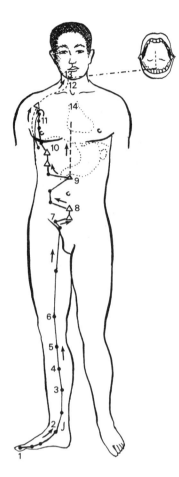

■ The Spleen Channel of the Foot—
Greater Yin (Zu Tai Yin Pi Jing)

■ The Heart Channel of
the Hand—Lesser Yin
(Shou Shao Yin Xin
Jing)

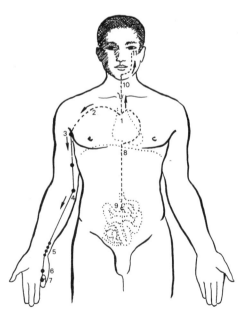

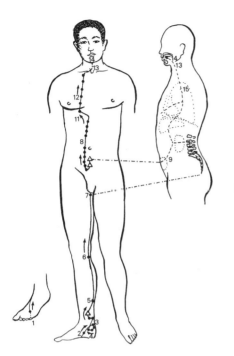

■ The Kidney Channel of the
Foot—Lesser Yin (Zu Shao
Yin Shen Jing)

■ The Pericardium Channel of
the Hand—Absolute Yin
(Shou Jue Yin Xin Bao Luo
Jing)

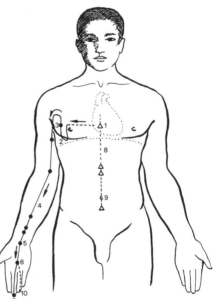

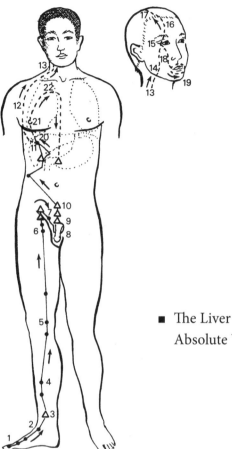

■ The Liver Channel of the Foot—
Absolute Yin (Zu Jue Yin Gan Jing)

5. There are thousands of secondary channels branching out from each primary channel; these lead the qi to the surface of the skin and to the bone marrow. It is very similar to the artery and capillary system. Instead of blood, qi is being distributed.

6. There are thirty-eight miscellaneous cavities on the sides of the vertebrae where the nerves branch out from the spinal cord (see illustration above). Stimulating these cavities properly can relax all the nerve junctions and also affect the qi circulation in the governing vessel.

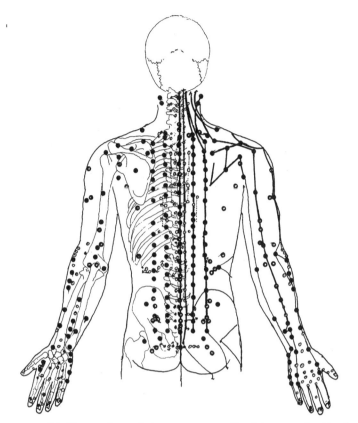

- Primary Qi Channels and Acupuncture Cavities on the Back of the Body

7. On each side of these cavities are two branches to the yang urinary bladder channel. This channel runs straight down from the top of the head to the bottom of the feet, splitting into two parallel branches on the back. On the inner branch are cavities that are closely related to the health of the internal organs.

For the purposes of this book, you do not have to remember all of these cavities and where they are located. Please refer to a book about acupuncture if you are interested in knowing more about these systems.

# Understanding the Central Energy System

1. The spine is the center of our qi distribution system. From the spinal cord, through the nervous system that branches out to the entire body, we can feel and sense our body and its surroundings. Moreover, through this system, our mind is able to govern and control our body for any activity.

2. The spinal cord is part of the thrusting vessel in Chinese medicine and connects the brain to the perineum. The qi in this vessel is most activated in the midnight hours, while we are sleeping. This vessel is connected directly to the qi residence or bioelectric battery, the "real lower dan tian," located at the physical body's center of gravity.

3. We actually have two brains. One is in our head and the other is in our gut. These two brains are connected with the spinal cord and communicate with each other. The spinal cord is a highly electric conductive tissue (having very low electric resistance). Therefore, even though physically there are two brains, they function as a single unit. The upper brain generates an idea—a form of electromotive force—and immediately the bioelectricity is supplied from the real lower dan tian through the nervous system to the part of the body that will be involved in action.

4. Whenever there is a tightness or strain in the spine, the qi distribution will be affected and could stagnate. Consequently, the nervous system will not function smoothly and efficiently. This means that communication between our brains and body will be slow or incomplete.

5. In order to have a smooth qi supply to the nervous system, the spine must maintain its comfortable and healthy state. All of this depends on the health and strength of your torso's muscles, which support the spine. When these muscles are weak or

injured, the pressure on the joints of the spine will be increased, resulting in back pain.

6. Due to the abundant qi supply circulating in the thrusting and governing vessels, most of our blood cells are produced in the bone marrow of our spine and pelvic bones. White blood cells are the soldiers of our immune system. When there are plenty of healthy white blood cells, our immune system is strong and defensive capability is high. Moreover, when the qi is abundant, each white blood cell will have the strength and power to destroy germs, bacteria, and other unwelcome material intruding into our body. Qi is just like the food for the soldiers. If soldiers do not have plenty of food, their fighting capability will be low. Therefore, the most important key to strengthening our immune system is to keep this central energy system healthy, both physically and energetically.

7. In the entire torso, the muscles' condition in the lower back area is the most important. This is the only area where there is no strong support from the skeleton. The only skeletal support in this area is the lumbar vertebrae; this allows us to bow forward and bend sideways and backward slightly. But the muscles in the lower back play an especially important role in supporting this area. When these muscles are injured or weak due to degeneration, the pressure on the lumbar vertebrae will be increased and pain will be generated. Therefore, in order to prevent lower back pain, the muscles in the waist area must be in good condition.

8. According to Chinese medicine, the kidney qi channel runs from the kidneys through the lower back to the bottom of the foot. Whenever there is a tightness or pain in the lower back, the qi status in the kidneys will be irregular—either too yin or too yang. When this happens, the function of the kidneys will

be abnormal. A common problem as a person ages is lower back pain is often followed by kidney problems.

9. From the perspective of both Western and Eastern medicine, we know that whenever we eat, after the blood absorbs nutrients in the large and small intestines, the blood then passes through the liver. The liver, like a check point, will filter the blood before the nutrients are distributed to the entire body through the circulatory system. During this process, acid is produced in the liver. This acid is then generally processed through the kidneys to the urinary system. That is why, when you get a physical, the doctor checks the pH value in your urine to see if the acid is being taken away from your body normally. If the kidneys fail or are functioning under some sort of stress, the acid level in the body will rise. This acid will normally accumulate in the joints and become the well-known form of arthritis called gout. Naturally, the qi level in the liver will also become abnormal, causing increased susceptibility to sickness.

10. According to Chinese medicine, the liver's condition is closely related to the heart. Whenever the qi is too yang in the liver, the heart will also become more yang. Too much yang in the heart can trigger a heart attack.

From the above discussion, you may already begin to see that the first and most essential key to maintaining health is to keep the torso strong, especially in the waist area. Next, you must know how to exercise the ligaments that connect the vertebrae joints. When these ligaments are strong and healthy, the spine is healthy. Spinal qigong exercise is one of the martial qigong practices that can lead you to this goal. In chapter 6, we will introduce these exercises.

# 2-3. Anatomical Structure of Our Back

In this next section, we will summarize the physical anatomical structure of our back. This synthesis of Western physical science and Eastern bioenergetic science will provide a more complete paradigm from which to analyze the factors that can affect your lower back.

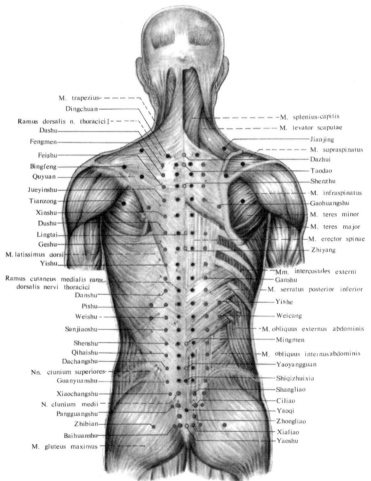

- Superficial Anatomical Structure of the Posterior Aspect of the Trunk

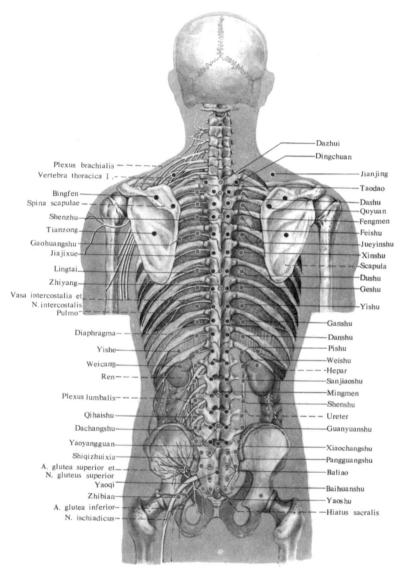

■ Deep Anatomical Structure of the Posterior Aspect of the Trunk

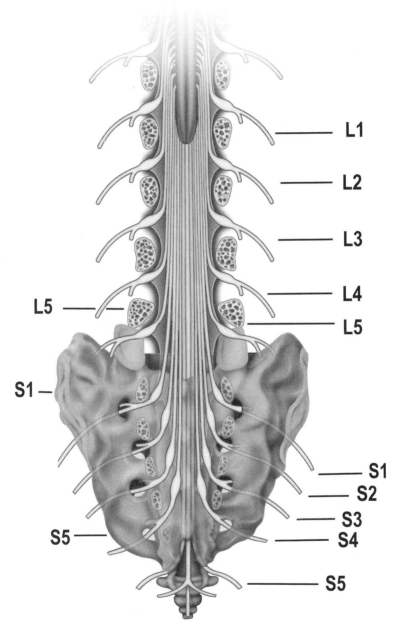

L1

L2

L3

L4

L5

L5

L5

S1

S1

S2

S3

S4

S5

S5

■ Nerve Distribution from the Spinal Cord to the Limbs
(Illustration by Shutterstock/Alexusmedical)

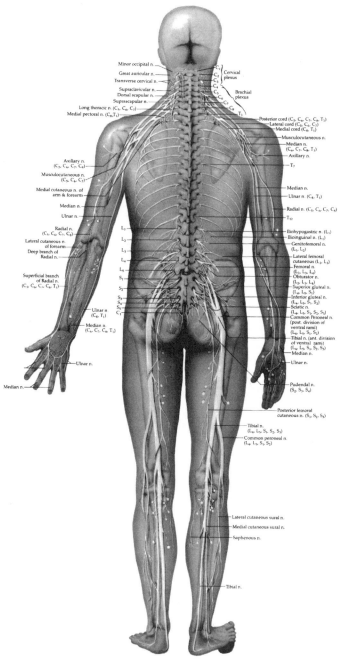

- **Nerves Branch Out (PNS) from the Spinal Cord (CNS)**
  (© Anatomical Chart Co., Skokie, IL)

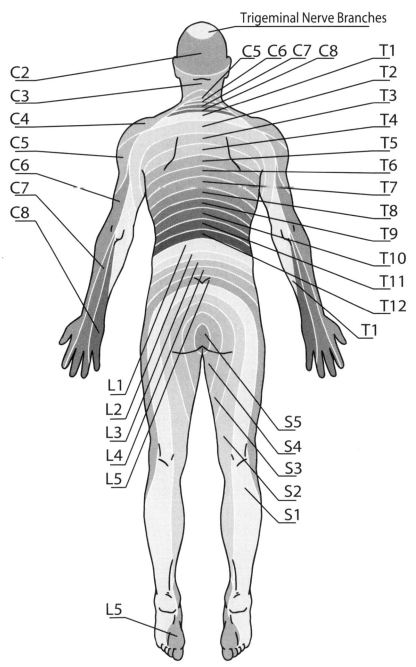

Trigeminal Nerve Branches

C5 C6 C7 C8 T1
C2          T2
C3          T3
C4          T4
C5          T5
C6          T6
C7          T7
C8          T8
            T9
            T10
            T11
            T12
            T1

L1
L2
L3          S5
L4          S4
L5          S3
            S2
            S1

L5

■ Dermatomes of the Upper and Lower Limbs
(Illustration by Shutterstock/stihii)

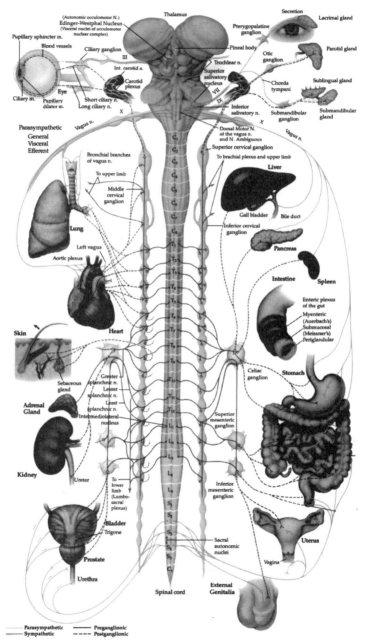

- A Schematic Representation of the Autonomic Nervous System and the Organs It Serves

(© Anatomical Chart Co., Skokie, IL)

Underneath the skin of our back, there are many sets of muscles. These muscles allow us to move our body. We can also see many nerve endings emerging from the muscles and spreading from the center to the sides (first illustration). Beneath the muscles are the spine and the ribs (second illustration). Most importantly, the peripheral nervous system (PNS) branches out from the spinal cord (third illustration). The nerves branch out from the spinal cord to the arms through the cervical and thoracic vertebrae, whereas the nerves from the lower portion of the spinal cord extend to the hips and legs through the lumbar vertebrae and sacrum (fourth and fifth illustrations). In addition, almost all of the nerves branching out from the spinal cord connect to various sensory organs and viscera, especially the nerves in the area of the thoracic vertebrae (sixth illustration). It is from these connections that our brain is able to sense our entire body and control it. Whenever there is a problem at any vertebra, this corresponding organ or area of the body will neither send nor receive clear impulses from the brain. We frequently perceive such a disturbance as pain. Often, we don't even perceive the disturbance until there is pain. Therefore, the physical health of your spine is one of the most important and critical requirements for your health.

Next, we will discuss the general structure of the spine. We will then review the nervous system in the back. Finally, because most back problems occur in the lower back, we will briefly summarize the structure of the lower back area.

# About the Spine

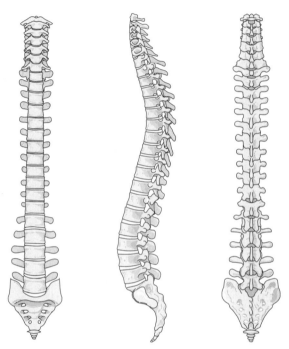

- Anterior View, Left Lateral View, and Posterior View of the Spinal Column
  (© *LifeArt Collection of Images,* Columbus, OH)

The spine is an extremely complex and elegant structure, made up of vertebrae, discs, the spinal cord, and nerves. Although we are born with thirty-three separate vertebrae, by adulthood most of us have only twenty-four. The nine vertebrae at the base of the spine grow together. The upper five of these nine lower vertebrae form a triangular bone and become the sacrum. The lowest four form the tailbone or coccyx and often fuse with the sacrum (see illustration above).

Physicians use a code to identify the vertebrae. The seven in the neck—the cervical vertebrae that support and provide movement for the head—are called C1 to C7. The thoracic vertebrae, numbered T1 to T12, join with and are supported by the ribs, which protect the heart and lungs. Because they are fairly rigid, thoracic vertebrae don't permit much movement and consequently are not injured as often as the other vertebrae. The lumbar vertebrae, numbered L1 to L5, are located below the thoracic vertebrae and above the sacrum. These are most frequently involved in back pain, mainly because they carry most of the body's weight and stress.

The vertebrae are not stacked one on top of the other in a straight line. Each rests on the one below at an angle, forming an S-curve when viewed from the side. The vertebrae would collapse

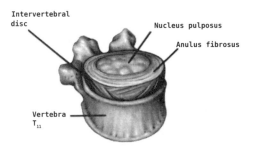

■ Spinal Disc
(© Anatomical Chart Co., Skokie, IL)

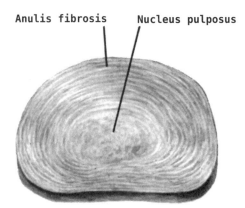

■ Structure of the Intervertebral Disc
(Frank H. Netter, M.D. *The Ciba Collection of Medical Illustrations,* *vol. 1, The Nervous System,* © 1983 Novartis)

without the tough ligaments that secure them together and the strong muscles and tendons that keep the spinal column upright.

Sandwiched between each pair of adjacent vertebrae is a spinal disc, twenty-three in all. Discs are flat, round structures (about one-quarter to three-quarters of an inch thick) composed of tough, fibrous outer rings of tissue that contain a soft, white jelly-like center. They actually grow larger at night. While we are resting, they absorb fluid from surrounding tissues. During the day, when we are active, the weight of the spine causes some of this fluid to ooze out, making us all a little bit shorter at the end of the day.

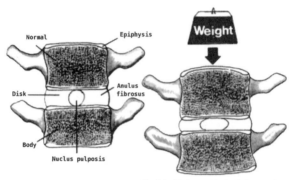

The disk with its contained gelatinous nucleus pulposus serves a cushioning purpose.

■ Function of Intervertebral Disc

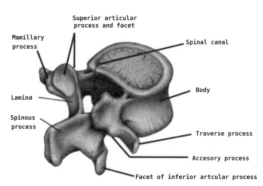

■ Structure of the Spinal Joint (Second Lumbar Vertebra)
(© Anatomical Chart Co., Skokie, IL)

Each disc is connected to the vertebrae above and below it by flat circular plates of cartilage. These flexible, flat pads not only keep the vertebra apart but also act as cushions between the hard bones. They compress when weight is put on them, and spring back when the weight is removed. Just like a car's shock absorbers, discs can degenerate from excessive stress or from just the wear and tear of daily life. But unlike a car's shocks, the cushiony discs cannot be replaced in kind.

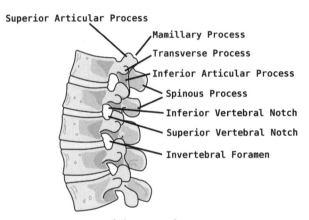

Superior Articular Process
Mamillary Process
Transverse Process
Inferior Articular Process
Spinous Process
Inferior Vertebral Notch
Superior Vertebral Notch
Invertebral Foramen

■ Connecting Structure of the Vertebrae
(© LifeArt Collection of Images, Columbus, OH)

While we need the strong, solid parts of the lumbar vertebrae to bear the body's weight, only joints will allow us to bend forward and backward, or to twist and turn. These joints are found in a ringlike structure of bone, known as the arch, located at the rear of each vertebra. The arch has a hollow center and little bones that go off in several directions, serving as anchors for muscles and ligaments. A pair of vertical bones projecting upward and another pair projecting downward—the facet joints—glide on similar smooth-surfaced bones in the vertebrae above and below them, creating an interlocking column of bones (see illustration above). The hollow areas of the arches form a channel (spinal canal) that encloses and protects the spinal cord. The only parts of the spine that we can feel with our fingers are projections from the bony rings called spinous (thornlike) processes. Each spinous process bends down slightly over the one below it to form an extra shield for the spinal cord.

The spinal cord, an extension of the brain, extends as far down

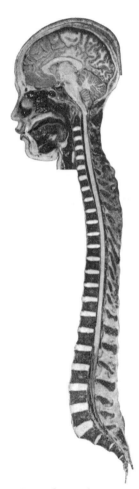

as L1, where it ends in a sheaf of nerves (cauda equina) resembling a horse's tail (see left illustration). Throughout the length of the spine, thirty-one pairs of nerves branch off from the spinal cord to serve all parts of the body, transmitting sensory messages to the brain (e.g., the water is cold) and messages from the brain to the muscles (e.g., "Lift your arm"). (See right illustration.) Where the nerves exit from the spinal cord through spaces (foramina) between adjacent vertebrae, they are called nerve roots. Few people are aware that if the neck is bent forward as far as it will go, the whole spinal cord moves upward in the spinal canal. Anything that prevents the cord and nerves from moving freely, such as abnormal bone growth within the spinal canal, will cause tingling or pain.

The 33 vertebrae, 23 discs, 31 pairs of spinal nerves, 140 muscles that hook onto the vertebrae, plus ligaments, tendons, and cartilage are all very complicated and all potential sources of back trouble. Small wonder that in 80 percent of cases,

■ Spinal Cord Extending from the Brain to Tailbone

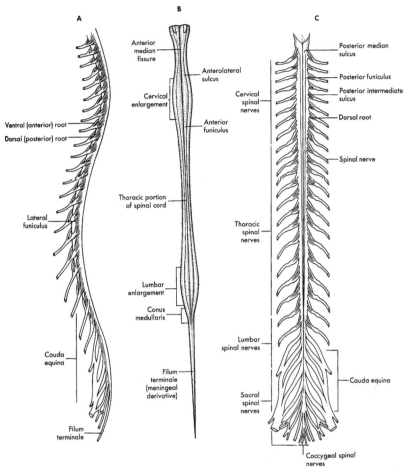

A

B

C

Anterior median fissure

Anterolateral sulcus

Cervical enlargement

Ventral (anterior) root

Dorsal (posterior) root

Anterior funiculus

Lateral funiculus

Thoracic portion of spinal cord

Lumbar enlargement

Conus medullaris

Cauda equina

Filum terminale (meningeal derivative)

Filum terminale

Posterior median sulcus

Posterior funiculus

Posterior intermediate sulcus

Cervical spinal nerves

Dorsal root

Spinal nerve

Thoracic spinal nerves

Lumbar spinal nerves

Cauda equina

Sacral spinal nerves

Coccygeal spinal nerves

■ Pairs of Nerves Branch Off from the Spinal Cord
(J. Robert McClintic, *Human Anatomy,* St. Louis, 1983, Mosby-Year Book, Inc.)

doctors cannot pinpoint the exact cause of back pain. Next, let us look at the nervous system in our back.

# The Nervous System in the Back

A nerve is a bundle of fibers joining the central nervous system to the organs and other parts of the body. Nerves relay sensory stimuli as well as motor impulses from different parts of the body to one another.

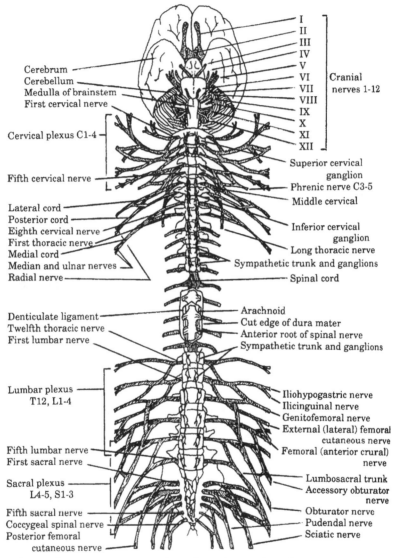

Cerebrum
Cerebellum
Medulla of brainstem
First cervical nerve

Cervical plexus C1-4

Fifth cervical nerve

Lateral cord
Posterior cord
Eighth cervical nerve
First thoracic nerve
Medial cord
Median and ulnar nerves
Radial nerve

Denticulate ligament
Twelfth thoracic nerve
First lumbar nerve

Lumbar plexus
    T12, L1-4

Fifth lumbar nerve
First sacral nerve

Sacral plexus
    L4-5, S1-3

Fifth sacral nerve
Coccygeal spinal nerve
Posterior femoral
    cutaneous nerve

I
II
III
IV
V
VI          Cranial
VII         nerves 1-12
VIII
IX
X
XI
XII

Superior cervical
        ganglion
Phrenic nerve C3-5
Middle cervical

Inferior cervical
        ganglion
Long thoracic nerve
Sympathetic trunk and ganglions
Spinal cord

Arachnoid
Cut edge of dura mater
Anterior root of spinal nerve
Sympathetic trunk and ganglions

Iliohypogastric nerve
Ilicinguinal nerve
Genitofemoral nerve
External (lateral) femoral
        cutaneous nerve
Femoral (anterior crural)
        nerve
Lumbosacral trunk
Accessory obturator
        nerve
Obturator nerve
Pudendal nerve
Sciatic nerve

- **Central Nervous System (CNS) and Peripheral Nervous System (PNS)**

All multicellular animals except sponges possess nervous systems. They are essentially regulatory mechanisms, controlling internal bodily functions and responses to external stimuli. The human nervous system is made up of two component subsystems: the central nervous system (CNS) and the peripheral nervous system (PNS).

Making up the CNS are the brain and the spinal cord, which are contained and protected within the skull and the spine, respectively. The CNS integrates, interprets, and transmits messages to and from the brain and the periphery of the body.

Making up the PNS is all the nerve tissue found outside of the skull and spinal column, including not only the nerve fibers that carry impulses but also groupings of fibers (plexuses) and nerve cell bodies (ganglions) that are found in the periphery. The PNS registers changes in internal and external environments of the body, transmitting this information to the CNS for action, and then delivering the orders of the CNS to muscles and glands for a response.

The PNS includes twelve pairs of cranial nerves that attach to the brain and their associated ganglions, as well as thirty-one pairs of spinal nerves and their ganglions. Finally, the PNS also includes specialized receptors and endings on muscles.

In terms of the function and interaction of all these constituent components, the PNS is simple and efficient. It is "built" out of somatic fibers (somatic nervous system) that provide the nerves for the skeletal muscles as well as the skin's special receptors (for touch, pressure, heat, cold) and autonomic fibers (autonomic nervous system). The autonomic fibers carry impulses to cardiac muscles and glands and from visceral receptors. These fibers make possible the reflexes that control breathing, heart rate, blood pressure, and other bodily functions in an involuntary and unbroken manner. Most organs receive fibers from two subdivisions of the autonomic nervous system. The parasympathetic (craniosacral) division is comprised of certain cranial nerves and several of the sacral spinal nerves.

It is responsible for many of the body's functions when at rest. The sympathetic (thoracolumbar) division is comprised of the thoracic and lumbar spinal nerves. This division furnishes impulses for the purpose of elevating body activity in order to tolerate or resist stressful or hazardous situations. In this way, an organ may have its operation intensified or diminished according to the demands of a survival situation.

This brief anatomical discussion of the nervous system shows us that the brain and spinal cord are the center of our feeling and functioning. We have seen that nerves from the spinal cord extend out and connect to the entire body, including the limbs and also the internal organs.

There are a number of other facts about the nervous system that are also important. First, our state of mind is linked to the condition of our physical body through our nervous system. This means that if we are mentally tense or relaxed, our physical body will react accordingly. Second, the nervous system is constructed of fibrous tissues, which are part of the material side of our body. In order to function properly, or even to stay alive, this material needs qi (bioelectricity). Third, if we compare the system of qi distribution to the nervous system, we see that although they are related, they are not the same system. The qi circulatory system does not only supply qi to the nervous system, but it also supplies it to all of the body's cells.

The nervous system plays a critical role in the practice of qigong healing for lower back pain. The nervous system enables us to feel what is going on everywhere in our body. Because the mind leads the qi, if we want to lead qi somewhere, we have to be able to feel that place. If we cannot feel that place, then the mind cannot lead the qi there because it has no reference to act as a guide.

The nervous system is responsible for our ability to feel, and it is our ability to feel that governs the qi. This means that the condition of the nervous system is directly related to the qi circulation in our body. Therefore, while in qigong healing we should pay particular attention to the qi system, the nervous system should be a close second in our priorities.

Because most back problems occur in the lower back, it is essential for us to understand the anatomy of the lumbar spine. The more we can understand this structure, the better we can envision the condition of our lower back and devise a way to correct any problems.

# Anatomical Structure of the Low Back (Lumbar) Spine

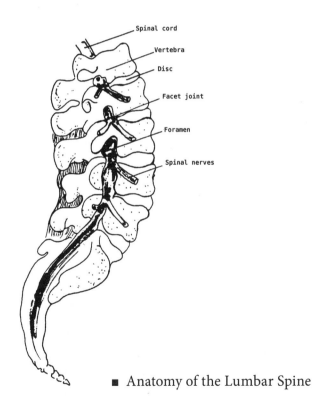

Spinal cord

Vertebra

Disc

Facet joint

Foramen

Spinal nerves

■ Anatomy of the Lumbar Spine

There are normally five lumbar vertebrae (see illustration above). The lumbar vertebral bodies are the largest of the vertebrae because of their weight-bearing functions. The vertebrae have both facet and intervertebral joints. The inferior facet joint from the vertebra above and the superior facet joint from the vertebra below form the facet joint. These joints are diarthrodial with synovial linings. That means that they permit relatively free movement. The intervertebral joints (between the vertebral bodies) are amphiarthrodial, a type of cartilaginous joint allowing little motion. These joints contain fibrocartilaginous discs consisting of avascular nucleus pulposus surrounded by annulus fibrosus. As explained earlier, the disc acts as a shock absorber, dissipating mechanical stress.

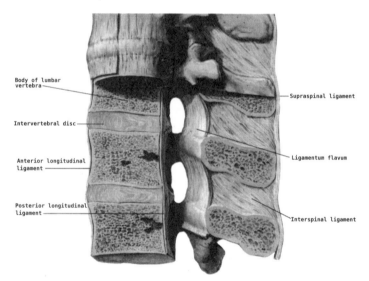

Body of lumbar vertebra

Intervertebral disc

Anterior longitudinal ligament

Posterior longitudinal ligament

Supraspinal ligament

Ligamentum flavum

Interspinal ligament

■ Ligaments of the Spinal Column

The vertebrae are surrounded by five different groups of ligaments that support and strengthen the spine (see illustration above). The lumbar vertebrae contain the spinal nerves, which exit at each level between the vertebrae through the neural foramen. The sinu-vertebral nerve is the major sensory nerve serving the structures of the lumbar spine.

Lumbar arteries arising from the aorta supply the vertebrae and ligaments with blood. The discs have no active blood supply and receive nourishment from the transfer of tissue fluid across the end plates of the disc by mechanical means. Three muscle groups support and move the lumbar spine. The erector spinae are the prominent paraspinal muscles of the lumbar spine. These muscles, in combination with the interspinales (muscles that run parallel to the spine), extend the lumbar spine. The abdominal and iliopsoas provide bending actuation (i.e., flexion).

# What Are the Possible Causes of Back Pain?

## 3-1. Introduction

Back pain can be caused by an overstretching of, other trauma to, the back muscles or tendons. It can also be caused by a tearing or inflammation of the ligaments in the spine. However, the most common and serious cause of back pain is spasm of the muscles in the lower back area brought on by spinal disease, injury, or degeneration. Naturally, all of these problems can arise from many different circumstances. In this chapter, we will summarize the possible causes in Western terminology. Because lower back pain is the most common type of back pain, most of the research materials I have collected focus on this area.

## 3-2. The Possible Causes of Back Pain

In order to have a clear understanding about lower back pain, we can envision the spinal elements structured as a "three-joint complex," with a disc and two facet joints at each level. If there are any changes in one element, the other two will also be affected. When a person assumes a normal relaxed, standing position, the vertebral bodies will be loosely piled up on top of each other. Whenever there is a disease that affects any one of the three elements, the intrinsic muscles will contract and develop protective splinting to prevent any microinstability that may occur. This can result in ischemia from prolonged contraction, and the muscles can begin to ache, lose tone, and eventually atrophy.

# Types of Pain

The prime symptom of spine problems is pain. Pain is the most common signal the body uses to notify your brain about the problem of qi imbalance or possible physical damage to your body. Pain generated from structures other than the spinal cord or nerve roots can be classified as local, referred, and muscular. If you are able to identify the type of pain you have, you may be able to better pinpoint the problem.

### Local Pain

Local pain usually results from the irritation of nerve endings at the site of the pathologic process. It is usually steady and aching and may occur off and on, particularly when the involved structure is moved. Local pain is commonly associated with tenderness to palpation or percussion. The site of local pain can be diagnosed relatively easier than other causes of back pain.

For example, metastatic tumors and osteoporotic collapse of a vertebral body can cause pain at the site of the lesion by irritating the nerve endings in the periosteum surrounding the vertebrae body. However, those metastatic tumors involving the vertebral body that do not upset the periosteum are usually painless. Other than the neck and lower back, tumors also often strike the thoracic area, and osteoporotic vertebral collapse also tends to affect the structurally weak thoracic vertebral bodies.

Intervertebral discs may also cause local pain when they compress nerve endings in the anulus fibrosus or posterior longitudinal ligament. Most spine pain from mechanical causes, such as a herniated disc, occur either in the neck or lower back because these structures are more mobile and more subject to injury.

The character of local pain is frequently helpful in diagnosis. Pain caused by lumbar muscle, ligamentous strain, or herniated discs usually disappears when the patient lies down and the torso is relaxed. Herniated lumbar disc pain is often made worse by sitting and is relieved when standing or walking. However, on the contrary, the pain of spinal stenosis is often absent when lying or sitting and occurs only when the patient walks. Vertebral metastases with or without epidural spinal cord compression cause pain. The pain is often more serious when lying and sometimes is relieved by sitting up. To ease the pain, many patients with spinal cord compression elect to sleep in a sitting position. Often, even if pain is absent when lying down, any movement such as turning over or arising may be particularly painful.

## Referred Pain, Radicular Pain, and Funicular Pain

**Referred Pain.** Referred pain is felt at a distance from the site of the local lesion but not in the dermatomal distribution of a nerve root (radicular pain). Referred pain, like local pain, has a deep, aching quality and is often associated with tenderness of subcutaneous tissues and muscles at the site of referral. Treatments for local pain usually have the same effect on referred pain. Referred pain produces a sclerotomal distribution of pain.[1] Pain referred from pathologic abnormalities of the cervical spine often is either just medial to the scapula or over the lateral aspect of the arm. Pain referred from the lower back is usually felt in the buttocks and posterior thighs, although rarely below the knees. Pain from the upper lumbar spine is also often referred to the flank, groin, and anterior thigh. Pain also can be referred to the spine from lesions of thoracic or abdominal viscera, a prominent example being back pain from pancreatic carcinoma. Referred back pain from a visceral source is usually not worsened by positional changes, as is mechanical lower back pain.

**Radicular Pain.** Injured spinal roots or an injured spinal cord can also produce, respectively, radicular or funicular pain. Radicular pain is the prime symptom of nerve root compression. Nerve roots are not usually pain-sensitive. However, chronic compression can lead to edema and perhaps inflammation and demyclination. In this case, the root will become sensitive to stretching or compression. When compressed, the pain may be experienced only in the cutaneous distribution (dermatome) of the involved root or may be felt locally and deep in muscles that it supplies. Root pain is usually least severe in proper positions in which the root compression is minimized. Naturally, the pain will become serious in positions that cause the root to be compressed or stretched. Root pain is usually worsened by increased intraspinal pressure due to coughing, sneezing, and straining.

Although similar, the pain distribution of radicular pain is not identical to referred pain. A common misconception is that referred pain radiates only as far down as the knee, and radicular pain radiates only below the knee. In fact, the only distinguishing feature between the two types of pain is in their quality. Referred pain is an aching or sore type of pain, while radicular pain is a sharp, lancinating, or burning type of pain.

Although the exact mechanism of nerve root compromise is not known, there are four known possible causes of radicular pain:

1.  Direct mechanical compression of the nerve (neuritis).

2.  Compression of the vasa nervorum, which produces a local anemia caused by mechanical obstruction of the blood supply (ischemia).

3.  Venous obstruction.

4.  Chemical irritation of the dural sleeve (i.e., the dura mater that covers the spinal cord), which causes inflammation (duritis). Dura mater is a tough, fibrous, whitish membrane (the outer-

most of the three membranes) that covers the brain and spinal cord.

**Funicular Pain.**[2] Funicular pain is caused by compression of the long tracts of the spinal cord. Normally, funicular pain is less sharp than radicular pain and is often described as a cold, unpleasant sensation in the extremity. Its distribution is more diffuse than that of radicular pain, but like root pain, it is usually worsened by movements that stretch the cord (e.g., neck flexion or straight leg raising) or that increase intraspinal pressure.

## Muscle Pain

Muscle pain occurs when paravertebral muscle spasm occurs due to an injury or to structural abnormality of the spine. Sustained contraction of paravertebral muscles causes chronic aching pain that is usually felt lateral to the midline of the neck or back. Palpation of painful muscles is a common diagnosis method to reveal evidence of spasm and tenderness. Often when areas of extreme sensitivity (trigger points) are palpated, the pain may be felt not only locally in the muscle but also may be referred to distant structures. These trigger points are considered to be the causes underlying many myofascial pain syndromes of the neck and back without structural abnormalities of the spine.

# Risk Factors

In the same environment, some people get sick more easily than others because their immune system is not as strong. Similarly, many people have a greater chance of developing back pain than others. The reasons for this are the "roots" of this type of pain. If you do not study these reasons but simply try to track down the causes of the symptoms, then even if you find relief, it is very likely that the problem will recur. Therefore, the best way of solving back pain problems and preventing them from occurring again is to find these roots. Next, we will examine the possible roots, or risk factors, that may cause back pain problems.

## Physical Degeneration[3]

We cannot stop our physical degeneration, but we can slow this degenerating process down by providing proper care to our body. According to Chinese qigong, to slow down our aging process, we must maintain the strength of our physical body (yang) and also learn how to increase the storage of inner energy in our qi body (yin). Normally, the health of our physical body can be achieved through physical exercises (physical qigong), and the storage of our qi in the lower dan tian (human bioelectric battery) can be obtained from correct breathing and meditation. When these yin and yang aspects of our body are cultivated, then health and longevity can be expected.

When we age, the first things to degenerate in our body are the muscles and tendons. Muscles reach their peak capacity by age twenty, then decline without proper exercise. When our muscles and tendons are degenerating and weakening, the body's motor capacity is going down. Consequently, the pressure between the joints of our body increases and the degeneration of the joints speeds up. This degeneration process is even greater in the spine, which supports our body's weight and activity.

The degeneration or deterioration of a part of the spine, especially the lower back, may result from a gradual wearing down of bone or soft connective tissue over time. It can also result from a reduction in the circulation of blood, which brings oxygen and other nutrients to the area. Degeneration is most likely to occur in the disc (cushion between the bones—vertebrae) or in the cartilage of the facet joints (joints between the vertebrae). In fact, both disc and joint disease are eventually present together.[1] "Degenerative lumbar spondylosis" refers to both. Therefore, degenerative disc disease can lead to degenerative joint disease and vice versa. When both the disc and the joint become involved, the pain is difficult to separate clinically.

Disc degeneration begins in the early twenties. Even though discs in babies are about 90 percent water, by age seventy, fluid loss reduces the water content to 70 percent, flattening the discs. Because discs constitute 25 percent of the spine's length, as the discs become flatter and less elastic, people lose height. In fact, most of us can expect to be about a half inch to two inches shorter in old age.

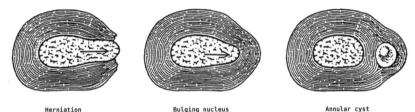

Herniation       Bulging nucleus       Annular cyst

■ The Nucleus Can Herniate or an Annular "Cyst" Can Bulge

In addition, when discs deteriorate, they can crack and slip outward (herniate), tear, or flatten, causing excessive movement and irritation of the cartilage at the facet joints. The nucleus pulposus changes into fibrocartilage from the second decade of life onward.[1] The loss of elasticity allows shearing forces to cross the disc unopposed. In addition, annular fibers can undergo localized myxomatous (degeneration caused by the presence of a benign tumor). This can lead to an osmotic gradient with the formation of a cyst within the annulus. This cyst can slowly enlarge and produce atraumatic disc bulging with consequent clinical signs and symptoms.

One or more discs might actually flatten, causing collapse of the vertebral column. When discs are flattened, they lose their ability to act as shock absorbers, putting greater stress on supporting ligaments, causing back pain. Pain can also result from the narrowing of the spinal canal (stenosis), which results in increased pressure on the nerves that branch out from the spinal cord.

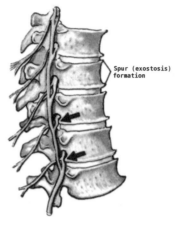

Spur (exostosis) formation

Arrows indicate bone spurs impinging on spinal nerves.

■ Spinal Nerve Irritation Due to Exostosis (Bony Overgrowth)
   (© Anatomical Chart Co., Skokie, IL)

In addition, as we age, various degrees of wear and tear on the spine may cause inflammation. This is commonly referred to as degenerative arthritis or spondylitis. If the degeneration is mild, no symptoms may appear. However, arthritis can destroy cartilage in the spine and cause bone overgrowth (spurs).

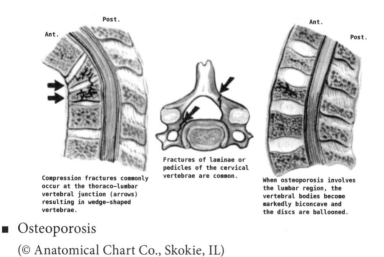

Compression fractures commonly occur at the thoraco-lumbar vertebral junction (arrows) resulting in wedge-shaped vertebrae.

Fractures of laminae or pedicles of the cervical vertebrae are common.

When osteoporosis involves the lumbar region, the vertebral bodies become markedly biconcave and the discs are ballooned.

■ Osteoporosis
   (© Anatomical Chart Co., Skokie, IL)

Another degenerative disease frequently affecting the back and causing back pain is osteoporosis. Osteoporosis is a condition in which bones become porous and susceptible to crushing or fracture. Even though both men and women lose bone density after age thirty-five, the disease appears most often in women past menopause.

Spinal joints are also affected by various forms of arthritis. One type that most of us will experience if we live long enough is degenerative joint disease, or osteoarthritis. The cartilage that cushions joints gradually breaks down, resulting in back pain and stiffness, especially in the morning. Osteoarthritis may appear as early as the twenties and thirties, though without symptoms, and nearly everybody has it by age seventy.

In many cases of arthritis, pain that begins in the morning upon arising from sleep improves throughout the day with activity. Because the nerves that branch out from the spinal cord conduct impulses to all parts of the body, pressure on one or more nerves may cause pain that radiates into the hip and down the leg (sciatica) or tingling or numbness of an arm or leg. In more serious cases, there may be interference with bowel and bladder function or, if nerves in the neck are compressed, difficulty speaking or respiratory problems.

Spinal osteophytosis, a normal function of aging, is produced by traction of the spinal ligaments on the periosteum of the vertebral bodies. It is not related to degenerative lumbar spondylosis.[1]

In spinal osteophytosis, the disc spaces are well preserved. The condition appears to be worse on the right side, probably due to inhibition of spur formation by the pulsating aorta along the left side. Approximately 90 percent of men older than fifty have some of these traction osteophytes in the lumbar area.

When spinal osteophytosis is excessive, it may represent a "forme fruste"—an atypical or incomplete form—of diffuse idiopathic skeletal hyperostosis (DISH), a predisposition toward ossification of the ligaments and tendons throughout the patient's body. DISH begins with ossification of the anterior longitudinal ligament of the dorsal spine and then spreads to the cervical and lumbar spine. It is associated with widespread osteoarthritis as well as spurs where the ligaments and tendons attach to bone (enthesopathy). DISH is typically found in middle-aged men, 80 percent of whom appear to have adult-onset diabetes. It is also seen as a side effect of isotretinoin (Accutane) and excessive fluorine intake.

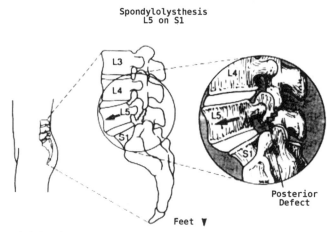

Spondylolysthesis
L5 on S1

L3

L4

L5

L4

L5

S1

Posterior
Defect

Feet ▼

■ Spondylolisthesis

Degenerative spondylolisthesis is a condition where there is a forward slippage of one vertebra over another, usually of a lumbar vertebra on the vertebra below it, or upon the sacrum. This condition is also called spondyloptosis. It is caused by subluxation, or slight misalignment, of degenerated joints. Spondylolisthesis almost always occurs at L4–L5.

From the above summary, we can see that the most common symptom of physical degeneration of the spine is an aching back. It is believed that failure to develop adequate bone mass during youth, lack of exercise, and a diet low in calcium and other nutrients (i.e., poor physical fitness) may be contributing factors.

## Poor Lifestyles

One of the most common and important root sources of sickness is the lifestyle we live. Unfortunately, this factor is greatly ignored by the general public until the start of a problem. If we look at Eastern and Western concepts of health, we can clearly see that one of their main differences is that Chinese medicine gives serious attention to the prevention of sickness, while Western medicine emphasizes healing after the symptoms of sickness appear physically. Qigong developed from the motivation to maintain health and longevity. It is also because of this that the Chinese have paid more attention to observing the relationship between natural qi and human qi. From this awareness, many qigong practices were initiated and blended into daily life. Since then, the ways of healthy living have been passed down from generation to generation for more than four thousand years.

If we calm down our mind, we can see a great difference between today's lifestyles and those of people living a century ago. Because of the fast development of science in this century, and despite the great benefits such development has brought us, our lifestyle has significantly changed and become less dependent on natural cycles, thus removing us from the natural Dao, or "way of life," to which our evolution has suited us. It is because of this new lifestyle, and the extremely short time in which we have had to adapt to it, that our body can have difficulties adapting to our environment. Therefore, many health problems can occur. The following are a few examples of such difficulties.

1.  The last fifty years have seen a rapid increase in cases of cancer. For example, it is estimated that 10 percent of women today will be diagnosed with breast cancer. If we analyze the reason, we may conclude that this may be a result of the heavy energetic and material pollution we have created in the last few decades. However, if we ponder more deeply, we can see that we

have ignored another important factor—our lifestyles have changed.

Traditionally, even just forty years ago, most women got married when they were young (often in their late teens). Due to lack of knowledge and poor reproductive medicine, on average women were pregnant at a younger age and more often than they are today. Normally, a woman would carry an average of ten babies in her lifetime.

Next, from a Chinese qigong and medical standpoint, we must understand that men are generally more muscular, bigger in size, and physically more powerful than women. There are only two places where a woman is normally larger than a man physically— the hips and breasts. The reason for this is that women have evolved bigger muscles in the hip area to support the baby's extra weight, and the bone structure of the pelvis is specialized for passing a child through the birth canal. Moreover, the breast area is more developed than in men because this place produces milk for the baby. In order to produce enough milk to nourish the baby, the qi in the breast area is normally highly abundant. From the baby's sucking of milk, the baby absorbs both nutrients and qi from the mother. Therefore, between mother and baby, there is a spiritual communication and a qi balance during this feeding process.

However, because we can now control reproduction, most women today will carry no more than two or three babies. Moreover, because of the convenience of bottle feeding, the spiritual communication and qi exchange process is missing. Therefore, there is a great quantity of underutilized qi stored in women's breasts today. If a woman does not practice qigong arm exercises correctly and lead the excess qi away from the breast area, the imbalance of qi in the breast may result in the physical deformity that is breast cancer. From a qigong point of view, this problem can become more significant because today's women do not exercise their arms as much as they used to. The arm exercises are the crucial keys of leading the accumulated qi away from the breast area. Furthermore, breastfeeding triggers increased hormone production and reduces breast cancer risk.

2.  It was reported in May 1996 that sperm counts in human males has been dropping significantly and steadily in the last two decades.[5] This implies that the human race could be facing a disastrous reproductive crisis in the not-so-far-off future. The data have been linked to a buildup in the environment of commonly used chemicals that some scientists believe disrupt the hormone systems controlling reproduction and development in humans.

However, again we have ignored the most important consideration: the change in our lifestyle. All human lifestyles in the past developed under the influence of nature. For example, before electricity was discovered, our sleeping habits were influenced by the sun's rising and setting. Normally, a person in ancient times would go to bed just a couple of hours after sunset and would wake up not long after sunrise. The qi circulation in our body has been significantly influenced by this natural cycle. During the day most of the qi was led by the mind to the muscles for daily physical activity (yang activity), while in the night, the physical body rested asleep, and the qi circulated inward to nourish the bone marrow, the brain, and the sexual organs through the spinal cord (i.e., thrusting vessel, yin activity).[6] Normally, this process and change from yang to yin takes about three hours, assuming deep physical rest and sleep. According to the understanding of Chinese qigong, the qi heavily and actively circulates in the central energy conduit (i.e., the spinal cord or thrusting vessel) at around midnight.

Now, let us take a look at today's lifestyle. Many of us these days do not go to bed until after midnight, which means we have already missed the natural timing of the brain's nourishment, as well as sperm production. This natural timing of sperm production has developed after millions of years of evolution. Naturally, it is not going to be easy to adjust to our new lifestyle in just a short few decades.

3. Today, we commonly experience more knee problems than we did forty years ago. What is surprising is that this has happened to both the young and the old. Human legs are much bigger and more powerful than arms, simply because we have walked for a million years by using our legs. After our body developed to this stage through walking, suddenly in the last forty years automobiles have become popular. We now travel by car almost everywhere, short trips as well as long. Walking from one place to another has become a painful process. Furthermore, due to today's flat roads, when we walk, we exercise only a specific set of muscles, tendons, and ligaments. That means the surrounding tissues around the ankles, knees, and hips are not used. This has caused the weakening of the joints area. Because of this, our legs have degenerated rapidly in the last forty years. A child spends many hours per week watching television or playing video games, then grows up to travel almost everywhere by car. Is it any wonder that our knees are not what they used to be?

4. Similarly, because of the absence of physical activity or exercise of our torso, our spine has rapidly undergone a general deterioration in the last few generations. This has resulted in increased spinal problems. Machines have replaced human labor to the benefit of many, but their use has also destroyed the natural body structure we evolved over millions of years.

In addition to the above four examples, there are many other problems caused by today's new lifestyle. Of course, I believe we should continue to develop science, technology, and medicine because of the wonderful benefits they bring to the world. However, the consequences of such developments are not without the potential for harm. We must pay more attention to these consequences as we consider what path our scientific development should take. For example, many kinds of electromagnetic radiation (radio waves, microwaves, etc.) pass through our body today at various levels of intensity. These human-made electromagnetic waves were nonexistent as recently as the beginning of this century. How do these waves affect our body? We have already discussed how our body, as a bioelectric organism, has an electromagnetic field that can be influenced by the surrounding electromagnetic field of the planet. How much will the energy circulating in our body be influenced because of the night shift—made possible by electric light—or even the time-dilating effects of jet lag? Therefore, we can see that it is our responsibility to urge our governments to give this area of study its proper attention. Only then will humanity really obtain the full benefits of its scientific development.

Now let us analyze and summarize the possible factors resulting from our current lifestyle that may be the causes of back pain.

**Imbalance of Torso.** Because the spine is a masterfully balanced piece of architecture, if there is an influence that is able to constantly disrupt the balance of our torso, the strain on one side of the torso can be worse than on the other side. Back pain can be caused as a consequence of this imbalance.

For example, shoes with high heels can make you constantly adjust your torso from leaning forward. This can generate imbalance-induced stress in the spine.

**Long Periods of Sitting or Standing.** It is believed that many cases of lower back pain are caused by stress in the muscles and ligaments that support the spine. Long periods of sitting and standing can make the torso muscles become fatigued and lose the strength to support the body's balance or upright posture. If a weak muscle is overburdened, it can go into spasm, affecting the whole network of back muscles. When this happens, back pain can result. This possibility is more significant for people whose physical fitness is poor. Often, even after the muscle spasm subsides, the muscle remains tighter than it was before the injury. This will limit movement in related joints and make new injury more likely.

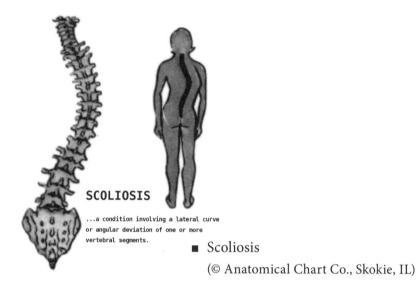

**SCOLIOSIS**

...a condition involving a lateral curve or angular deviation of one or more vertebral segments.

■ Scoliosis
(© Anatomical Chart Co., Skokie, IL)

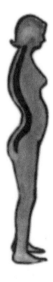

**LORDOSIS**

...an exaggeration of the posterior concavity of the spine characteristic of the lumbar region. It is also called "swayback" indicating extreme anterior curvature of the lumbar spine.

■ Lordosis
(© Anatomical Chart Co., Skokie, IL)

**Poor Postures or Improper Body Movements.** Habitual poor posture in sitting or standing can generate an imbalance in the torso. This will affect the structure of the spine. Normally, this problem can result from activities associated with poor posture, such as watching too much television, working for too long on a computer, or poor sleeping habits (i.e., on the stomach, on a soft mattress). Scoliosis or lordosis (see illustrations above) are common spine problems resulting from the uneven narrowing of one area of the discs. These problems can be exacerbated by poor posture.

Sometimes improper body movements can cause damage to the spine. For example, a sudden twist or fall can bring on muscle spasm (sudden, involuntary contractions that can be excruciatingly painful). A spasm immobilizes the muscles over the injured area, possibly acting as a kind of splint to protect muscles or joints from further damage. Improper body movements usually occur while you are engaged in physical labor or sports.

**Poor Physical Fitness.** If you are in poor physical condition, especially in the abdominal muscles, you cannot support the spine properly, and strain or sprain can be recurrent. The fact is, it doesn't take much to overstretch (strain) a muscle or put a small tear (sprain) in a ligament. The medical word for backaches arising from either of these conditions is lumbosacral strain (or sprain).

The main causes of poor physical conditioning are lack of exercise or improper exercise. Too little exercise results in a lack of strength in the torso. Too much exercise can also be harmful, especially when the muscles are in a fatigued condition and can be easily injured. Good exercise for healthy physical fitness is exercise that is able to build up both the strength and endurance of the muscles, tendons, and ligaments.

**Obesity.** Bad eating habits or poor food choices can cause obesity. This can worsen if the person also fails to exercise. Obesity increases both the weight supported by the spine and the pressure on the discs within the spine, therefore generating spine problem more often than in other people.

**Job-Related Stresses.** Jobs that involve bending and twisting or the lifting of heavy objects repeatedly, especially when the loads are beyond a worker's strength, are no better for the back than are sedentary jobs. Certain occupations, such as truck driving or nursing, are particularly hard on the back. The truck driver must contend with sitting for long periods (actually worse for the back than standing), the vibration of the vehicle, and lifting and straining at the end of the day when muscles are fatigued and more susceptible to damage. It has been shown that the dorsal muscles become easily fatigued when subjected to seated vibration.[7] In fact, truck driving ranks first in workmen's compensation cases for lower back pain.

**Sports or Gymnastics.** Football, gymnastics, and other strenuous sports can also damage the lower back. In addition, degeneration may also occur in younger people, such as ballet dancers or athletes, where required movements repeatedly place extreme pressure on one or more parts of the spine. A curvature of the spine (scoliosis) may cause the vertebral joints to move in abnormal ways, leading to more pronounced degeneration.

**Smoking.**[7] An 18 percent greater mean disc degeneration score in all levels of the lumbar spine has been reported in smokers as compared with nonsmokers. Overconsumption of alcohol may also be involved in disc degeneration.

# Genetic Predisposition

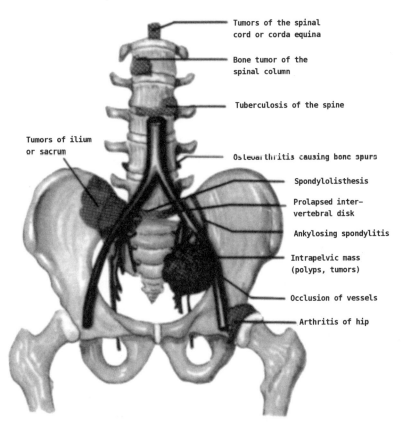

Tumors of the spinal
cord or corda equina

Bone tumor of the
spinal column

Tuberculosis of the spine

Tumors of ilium
or sacrum

Osteoarthritis causing bone spurs

Spondylolisthesis

Prolapsed inter-
vertebral disk

Ankylosing spondylitis

Intrapelvic mass
(polyps, tumors)

Occlusion of vessels

Arthritis of hip

Not all back pains are caused by protruding disks or extruded nucleus pulposis. Shown
above (diagrammatically) are ten other causes that the examining physician must
consider as possibilities in the diagnosis.

■ Ankylosing Spondylitis
(© Anatomical Chart Co., Skokie, IL)

A particularly distressing type of arthritis is ankylosing spondylitis (see illustration above). The lower back and sacroiliac joints
became stiff and swollen. Muscles spasm and back pain may be so
severe that bending over is the only way to find relief. If untreated, in
some cases the inflamed spinal joints may fuse, preventing the individual from straightening up. The disease affects more men than
women, usually starting between the ages of twenty and forty,

although it can begin as early as age ten. The cause is unknown, but it is believed that some people may be genetically susceptible to this disorder. Posture-maintaining exercises, hot baths, painkillers, and nonsteroidal anti-inflammatory drugs may help relieve symptoms.

In addition, those people whose height is above average can also experience back pain more frequently than those of average height. This is simply because it is harder for them to bend their upper body without putting more stress or strain on the lower back. The worst part of life for these overly tall people is using mass transportation, utilities, clothes, machines, and so forth, which are designed for people of average height. The necessity of living their life in a world two feet too short can be depressing, both mentally and physically.

It is also a fact that our two legs are normally not the same length. If the difference is over a quarter inch, the imbalance to the torso can cause muscle spasms, especially if you have to walk for a long distance.

## Mental (Spiritual) Excitement or Depression

Mental (spiritual) excitement or depression can occur if you are emotionally disturbed. For example, too much excitement or sadness can create strain in the torso and therefore cause back pain. Learning to regulate your mind and maintain your emotions in a neutral and harmonious state can have positive influences.

Another common factor in depression is work dissatisfaction. According to reports, individuals who stated that they "hardly ever" enjoyed their job tasks were 2.5 times more likely to report back injury than were those who "almost always" enjoyed their jobs.[7] When this happens, emotional depression can be generated, which could result in back pain.

# CHAPTER 4

# How Does Western Medicine Treat Back Pain?

## 4-1. Introduction

Before the development of modern medicine, when a person suffered back pain, it was treated with rest, massage, heat, or gentle movements until the pain subsided. When modern medicine became popular in the second half of the twentieth century, painkilling drugs, ice to reduce inflammation, and rest were heavily utilized. However, in recent years, as we have gained a better understanding of the anatomic structure of the spine and learned more about the possible causes of these problems, and as the price of clinical medical treatments has gone up, a new paradigm for treatment and experiments has emerged. Here are some of the facts that have been discovered by modern Western medicine according to recent reports.[1,2]

1. Back pain is one of the diseases that is most difficult for the physician to diagnose. It is often troublesome to treat and always lasts longer than patients and their caregivers would like.

2. Most back pain is caused by muscles that go into spasm. The cause of the spasm of the muscles can be either unrelated or closely related to spine problems.

3. The majority of back pain problems are self-correcting and resolve within a few weeks.

4. Lower back pain and disability do not progressively increase with age, nor does it correspond to the age-related changes of disc degeneration.

5. There is little difference in the effectiveness of any type of treatment for lower back pain, and there is no scientific evidence that any one treatment is any better than others.

6. Chronic lower back pain is a completely different syndrome than acute lower back pain and is treated differently.

7. According to a study in the *New England Journal of Medicine*, two days of bed rest are enough for most acute backaches. More than two days' rest can further weaken muscles.[3]

8. The traditional explanation for chronic back pain, the "slipped disc," actually accounts for less than 5 percent of back injuries. In fact, with the increased use of CT scans, doctors are now finding that many people, if not most, have disc abnormalities that don't contribute directly to pain.

9. Back pain is an overtested and often overtreated problem (imaging, surgery, medication), due in part to the fact that many research studies have not been well defined. Only about 1 percent of people with back pain require surgery. It is believed that there are almost twenty times more back operations per capita in the United States than Canada, and the fact is that this does not result in a greater treatment success rate. Surgery is definitely overdone.

In the next section, we will consider some suggestions from Western medicine for preventing back pain, and some important tips for posture will be provided in section 4-3.

# 4-2. Western Medical Treatments

Recently, a new concept of treatment has arisen and has been proven to work well, at least no worse than traditional methods. The trend is away from passive therapies and toward greater self-reliance and a return to activity as soon as feasible. A "wait and see" interval could turn into a period of deconditioning. The more patients can do on their own and the sooner they can do it, the greater the physical as well as psychological benefits.

Next, we would like to summarize the general treatments for back pain. In this summary, both conservative traditional methods and new techniques are included. Therefore, use your own judgment in selecting the method for your case. Remember, even today, we still cannot be sure which techniques are more effective than others. Naturally, you should also realize that the effectiveness of a treatment also depends on how the problem was started. The better you can pinpoint the problem from diagnosis, the easier you may solve the problem.

Before we summarize the treatments, there are a few initial suggestions from Western medicine to consider if you are stricken with back pain:

1. Wait for the discomfort to calm down before you begin to stimulate or actively move your back muscles.

2. Once you feel more comfortable, stay active if you can and, if possible, resume physical activity as soon as possible.

3. If the pain is extreme, use medications wisely and cautiously. Avoid narcotics if at all possible.

4. If you so desire, see a chiropractor once or twice. It may be a simple spinal alignment problem causing tension in the back muscles. Sometimes a chiropractor is able to correct the problem in a short time.

5. The last method is seeing a doctor and getting a physical. Most patients don't need X-rays. Often, a few simple questions will identify those who do.

## General Treatments[1,5]

**Short Period of Rest.** The most basic treatment for acute back pain is a short period of rest, no more than two days. In the past, one to two weeks of bed rest was recommended by physicians. However, a recent study has reported that resting longer than two days is not necessarily more effective than only two days of bed rest.[6,7] Moreover, while there is no firm scientific evidence to show that bed rest is beneficial, there is ample evidence for the deleterious effects of bed rest. In fact, there is a 3 percent loss of muscle strength per day during bed rest, resulting in decreased physical fitness. Prolonged rest can only lead to depression, loss of working habits, and difficulty in starting rehabilitation.

So far, there is no indication that activity is harmful or makes the pain worse in the long term. On the contrary, increased activity promises to promote bone and muscle strength and may also increase endorphin levels. People who keep physically fit are at less risk for episodes of back pain. Activity is not harmful, and active rehabilitation helps to restore function and reduce pain.

**Applications of Ice or Heat.** Application of ice or heat to the aching area is probably one of the most common treatments for any pain. In ice therapy, ice packs or ice massage is applied or rubbed over the painful area for fifteen minutes every hour or more; this can alleviate acute pain. If ice is applied, a towel should be placed over the skin to protect it.

Moist heat is an alternative to ice therapy. When heat is used, the patient can be more relaxed and feel more comfortable, and the blood circulation may improve. Consequently, pain and stiffness can be eased. In heat therapy, moist warm towels are used by themselves or in combination with a heating pad. In order to avoid burns and the generation of negative effects, heating pads should not be left on for more than thirty minutes.

**Medications.**[4] Often, medications are used to ease pain or reduce discomfort. However, you must recognize two important facts. First, medications can solve the symptoms only temporarily. Medications do not address the root of the problem. Once medication wears off, the discomfort will normally return. Second, almost all medications generate side effects. If you decide to take medications, you should consider all of these factors.

For nonprescription medicine, acetaminophen and ibuprofen can help relieve pain and swelling. There are also many medications that can help reduce discomfort. Narcotic analgesics can decrease discomfort. However, narcotics can cause constipation and depression, decrease function, and suppress natural endorphins.

One of the most common types of medication ordered is muscle relaxants, such as cyclobenzaprine (Flexeril), methocarbamol (Robaxin), or carisoprodol (Soma). There is little evidence to support their efficacy. The most common side effect of muscle relaxants is drowsiness.

Nonsteroidal anti-inflammatory medications (NSAIDs) are also commonly prescribed. These medications block prostaglandin production and reduce inflammation, thus helping reduce the pain. There are many side effects of their usage, including gastrointestinal distress, such as nausea, heartburn, and diarrhea; kidney impairment; and fluid retention. No one group of NSAIDs has proven more effective than any other group.[7] Failure with one NSAID does not mean others will be ineffective too. Short-term systemic corticosteroids are still occasionally prescribed, but it should be stressed that even short-term use may cause significant long-term side effects.

**Physical Therapy Modalities.** Physical therapy using TENS (transcutaneous electrical nerve stimulation) units, diathermy, ultrasonography, and hydrotherapy may be prescribed. They may reduce muscle spasms and pain temporarily. When used in combination with exercise, these methods may facilitate earlier mobilization and improve function. Controlled studies have yet to show the effectiveness of these modalities alone. In fact, a study at the Seattle Veterans Affairs Medical Center shows that stretching exercises are at least as effective at reducing pain as TENS.

**Exercises.** Today, experts estimate that between 70 to 90 percent of back pain is caused by muscle or ligament problems, usually related to weakness in the lower back, rather than by serious damage to the spine itself. It is also believed that most of the problems can be cleared up within a few weeks. However, if the strength of the lower back is not built up to a healthy level, most likely the pain will return. It is common for most doctors to treat the pain, not the underlying disorder that caused the pain. Consequently, when patients go back to their unchanged lifestyle, they end up hurting themselves again.[2]

In the late 1980s many Western medical scientists started to believe that the best cure for back pain and the prevention of relapse is to strengthen the back muscles through exercise. That means muscular rehabilitation. This new concept of treatment emphasizes not only treating the pain but also keeping the patient up and about as much as possible to avoid the debilitation that results from inactivity. Routine use of medications and invasive modalities is discouraged. Naturally, this was a revolutionary concept that differed from the traditional Western medical consensus that advised that the patient take medicine and then rest. Back treatment programs are now changing from traditional rest-and-drug therapy to a new approach of aggressive exercise.[1]

A variety of exercise programs have been developed to treat back pain, and the results have been significant. Some experts found that isometric exercises are the most effective.[8] Exercise should be started gradually and gently at first, increasing as the recovery process continues. Daily activities should also be encouraged because the increased activity will promote bone and muscle strength and also increase endorphin levels. In fact, there is no evidence that early return to work and its associated activities will increase the future recurrence of back pain. Patients should be urged to gradually increase their fitness levels. According to one report, those in the most physically fit group were ten times less likely to develop back ache than those in the least physically fit group.

**Corset or Brace.** Corsets and braces decrease motion in the lumbar spine but do not achieve complete immobilization. It has been found that there is more relief of back pain by a corset with spinal support than by one without such support.[9] Corsets increase intra-abdominal pressure and may decrease intradiscal pressure.[3] The primary disadvantage of brace usage is a loss of muscle function leading to local muscle weakness. An exercise program to maintain muscle function should therefore accompany brace usage.

**Manipulation.** The most controversial treatment for back pain is spinal manipulation. No clear-cut guidelines or indications exist for the use of manipulation. There is no clear understanding for how manipulation works. Manipulations are expected to increase mobility, readjust the vertebrae, reduce the size of disc herniations, reduce spasms, and, most of all, decrease pain. Short-term manipulation by chiropractors or osteopaths may temporarily decrease pain and improve function.[10] But when the problem is disc herniation or osteoporosis, manipulation may make matters worse.

**Back School.** One of the most important and effective components of back pain treatment is education.[11] Back school is a program that provides in-depth information about anatomy of the spine, exercises, and body mechanics to help individuals with back pain manage their symptoms and minimize future injury. This can best be done by a nurse or physician who understands the mechanisms of back pain and its medical management. Patients with back pain often have difficulty dealing with the pain, becoming discouraged by its effect on their daily lives and quality of living, and experiencing frustration with the medical community's inability to provide a cure. Through educational programs, patients can understand their condition and build up confidence in dealing with the problem, both physically and psychologically.

**Surgery.**[4] It was estimated in 1987 that fewer than 10 percent of the cases of lower back pain required surgery. Moreover, out of the surgeries performed, only about 75 percent really got great results. It is believed that often the wrong operation is done, or an operation is done on a patient who could have gotten by without one.

Although physicians prefer to treat even severe cases of lower back pain in a conservative manner with bed rest and painkillers, surgery is clearly called for if pressure on a nerve root causes severe pain lasting for weeks, or if progressive damage to the nerves results in leg weakness or paralysis. Every year, about two hundred thousand Americans undergo surgery for persistent back pain.

The most common surgery is the removal of the slipped or herniated disc. In this operation, the doctors get at the disc by removing only a very small part of the bone—the arch of the vertebra (this procedure is called a laminectomy). Then, they remove the part of the disc that is out of place and any other loose fragments that are accessible.

Another condition that requires laminectomy is spinal stenosis, an unusual narrowing of the space inside the spinal canal. A narrow spinal canal may cause pressure on the nerve roots and, in rare cases, on the cord itself. This is the second most common operation for back pain treatment. The reason for this necessity is that some people are born with a narrow spinal canal, while others develop a buildup of ligaments and bone spurs that also narrow the spinal canal. This results in wear and tear and having the spine work against gravity over time.

In some cases, spinal fusion is done. Because the spine is made up of a number of joints, and if a joint is unstable and slips, causing nerve root pinching, the slipping is stopped by fusing the two vertebrae together. To do this, surgeons insert fragments of the patient's own bone, usually taken from the hip, to bridge the space between two adjacent vertebrae. In time, the bones grow together. Fusion relieves pain but reduces mobility.

## Other Treatments[4]

Another technique called aspiration percutaneous lumbar discectomy (APLD) may be useful for those for whom general anesthesia is risky. Using x-ray pictures as a guide, the neurosurgeon or orthopedist inserts a long, thin needle called a nucleotome probe into the center of the protruding disc. The physician loosens the disc material by moving the probe back and forth. A pump that is attached to the probe suctions up the material and carries it away.

APLD takes about forty minutes, requires about ten days of recuperation, and costs a great deal less than laminectomy. However, not everybody is a suitable candidate for this procedure. It cannot be used on those who have severely ruptured discs or spinal stenosis.

# 4-3. Suggestions from Western Doctors

Because of our early education, we become convinced that pain means sickness. We do not recognize that pain is a signal from the body to inform the mind that we are doing something wrong, not necessarily that something is wrong. Often, instead of addressing the cause, we become pushovers for pills, driving the pain underground. Consequently, sickness is generated, and the condition continues to worsen. According to Chinese medicine and qigong, pain or any feeling of discomfort is actually the language that the body uses to communicate with the brain. If the brain does not register this message, serious and chronic problems will eventually manifest. One of the most important parts of Chinese qigong is learning how to feel the body's condition. This kind of training is called internal vision (i.e., internal feeling).

In this section, we will summarize a number of valuable suggestions and key tips from Western doctors for back pain prevention. These suggestions will not only help you correct the possibly already wrong lifestyle that you may have for future back pain but also provide you with a better awareness of and alertness to your body's signals or condition. Only when you have this awareness can you appreciate early warning signs of a problem and prevent it from getting worse.

## Suggestions[1]

**Educate yourself.** The most important method of preventing the occurrence of back pain is education. First, you should understand the anatomic structure of your back, especially the spine. Next, you must research the possible causes of back pain. Naturally, reading or studying other patient's experience can bring attention and awareness to your own situation.

If possible, try to understand the existing treatments. Because it is almost impossible to pinpoint the cause of back pain and the treatment effectiveness is often vague, it might be wise to examine and use both the Western and Eastern methods of treatment. Finally, you should study your lifestyle and analyze your body's condition, both physically and mentally. Only through these educational processes can you direct yourself to a healthy path of life.

**Use common sense.** Before you can use your common sense to take action, you must first build up a habit of awareness and alertness. Once you can bring yourself to attention, then you can analyze the situation and make a wise judgment. For example, often you are in a bad sitting posture while watching television. However, if you can bring awareness and thought to the situation, you can correct this mistake before any problem starts. Other examples: Do you use safe lifting and handling techniques and body mechanics? Does your workplace make you feel depressed or tensed?

Naturally, the more you are educated about the spine's structure and possible causes of pain, the better you can correct any problems. The key is to be aware of the body's condition and the activities involved. When you use your common sense to make judgments, you can avoid most unnecessary injuries or problems.

Later, we will list a few keys to spine protection from different situations and body postures.

**Stay physically fit.** The next important means to prevent back pain from occurring is to keep your body in a physically healthy condition. This includes the compact bone structure as well as the strength of the ligaments, tendons, and muscles. When these factors are strong, you will have a firm and solid foundation to keep your physical body in a balanced condition. When your body is in a balanced state, the torso posture will be correct, and the strains and stresses on the spine will be minimized.

The best way to keep this balance is to improve the strength of the back's extensor muscles, which allow you to uncurl from a tucked position and stand upright against gravity. When the extensors are weak, the pelvis tips forward, robbing the lower back of support, and the hamstring and hip muscles end up taking over most of the lower back's load. This creates tightness in the hamstrings and hips, and leaves the lower back chronically weak.[2]

Therefore, correct ways of exercising to maintain the health of the muscles and spine are important. With the correct exercises, those muscles that support the spine and reduce its strain will be strengthened. Wrong exercises may either cause back pain or worsen it. Moreover, you must also know that exercise and relaxation should mutually balance each other. Too much exercise can make your muscles fatigued and more strained or tightened. Too much resting will make the muscles degenerate and weaken.

In fact, the hardest part of maintaining physical strength is not learning exercises but maintaining a schedule of exercise. Often, we are conquered by our lazy mind and quit easily. Truly, it is our mind that makes our bodies both physically and mentally weak and degenerate. Therefore, the keys to preventing yourself from getting sick are learning to conquer yourself and establishing a healthy lifestyle.

**Reduce stress.** It is well known that emotional strain can cause the back muscle to tighten and therefore increase the stress on the spinal joints. Often, mental stress originates from an abnormal lifestyle, from mental anxiety, from an unhappy job environment, or from feelings of guilt. If this is the case, then you must first analyze and learn the cause of your stress and correct it. If this cause is not corrected, the problem will return.

In Western medicine, one of the possible treatments for tightened back muscles is to make the patient exercise in a pool while wearing a buoyant vest with weights suspended from the waist. The idea is to stretch the spine and attached muscles. This treatment has been reported to result in an 80 to 85 percent improvement among patients.[5]

Some machines, such as the MedX back and neck machine developed by Arthur Jones, inventor of the Nautilus weight machine, are able to hold the patient's pelvis down tight with restraining mechanisms controlled by a therapist. Once the lower body is immobilized, the patient, who is sitting in a tucked position, pushes backward with the upper body against preset resistance, working just the lower back muscles.

**Avoid or stop smoking.** According to statistical analysis, it is believed that there is a possible relationship between symptomatic disc disease, such as prolapsed lumbar disc and a prolapsed cervical disc of the spine, and cigarette smoking.[12] The fact is that most patients with symptomatic disc disease and a majority of the patients with acute lumbar disc herniation who undergo surgery are smokers. Theoretically, it is possible that smoking is related to decreased blood oxygenation to the disc, which interferes with the repair process of the body, specifically the disc, and thus it ages or degenerates prematurely. Smokers also cough more than nonsmokers, which increases the pounds of pressure on the disc, resulting in increased physical stress to the disc. Of course, in order to quit your smoking habit, you must first conquer yourself mentally.

**Avoid obesity.** To maintain your normal weight is one of the main keys to ensure that the trunk will not carry any additional physical load. Moreover, because of greater abdominal girth, an obese individual is normally a greater distance from the objects he or she is lifting. Furthermore, he or she may also have more difficulty squatting to lift. The fact is that the farther away an object is from the individual's center of gravity, the higher the risk for strain to the lower back.

# Important Tips for Body Postures

## Sitting

1. Avoid sitting in one place or in one position for a long time. Get up and stretch, walk about, and change positions. Bring your awareness and common sense into your consciousness. Often, placing a cushion or rolled-up towel under your back can help you feel more comfortable.

2. If you sit for a long time, rest your feet on a low stool. But do not generate more tension in the knee area, which may cause injury to the knees. Keep your knees bent.

3. Avoid sitting in soft, deep seats. If you are having back pain, try to sit in a chair with arms that will help you get up and down.

4.  At a desk or in the car, sit so your knees are level with your hips. This will reduce some of the stress on the lower back.

5.  When driving, adjust the seat so your legs don't have to stretch to reach the pedals. In addition, you should get out and stretch every twenty to thirty minutes. This will loosen your torso and reduce the strain on the lower back.

## Lifting[1]

1.  Think before moving. Again, this is an awareness of the conditions around you and use of your common sense to make a wise judgment.

2.  Clear the area of clutter. Before you lift, you should check around you and clear the space. This will allow you to have a better maneuvering area if you have problems with the lifting.

3.  Test the load. Before you lift, test it first. This will help you understand your capability and the potential for injury.

4.  Keep all lifted objects close to your body. When you lift, the closer the object is to you, the better balance you will have and, therefore, the less strain you will have on your back muscles.

5.  Use a wide, balanced stance like a weight lifter. In order to have good balance for your lifting, you should keep your legs apart and seek for the best balance and most comfortable position for your lifting.

6.  Avoid lifting anything while you are reaching, twisting, or bending forward. Also, you should avoid jerking while lifting.

7.  When lifting, bend your knees and use the force of your legs to help lift in a smooth motion. Don't bend over at the waist with your legs straight.

8.  Tighten the back and abdominal muscles. This will protect your ligaments and vertebrae and help prevent injury.

9. Don't lift a heavy load above your waist. It will definitely be worse if the height is above your chest.

10. Avoid lifting more than 35 percent of your body weight without help.

11. Use lumbar belts. Lumbar belts are used to prevent back muscle injuries. They do so by prohibiting poor lifting techniques and employing other muscles to perform the majority of the work. Be aware, though, that according to one study, belts do not increase the strength of the lower back muscles or help the wearer lift heavier weights.

## Sleeping

1. Use a firm mattress. Too soft or too rigid is not good for the back.

2. Find the sleeping position that is most comfortable. This may mean sleeping on your side with your knees bent, or on your back or side with a pillow under your knees, or not using a pillow at all.

3. Never sleep on your stomach. Sleeping on your stomach will not help your back pain problems. Sleeping this way will normally exaggerate your pain and often creates neck pain and headaches.

## Walking

1. Try to take a brisk walk every day. Be sure to wear comfortable, well-cushioned, low-heeled shoes.

2. Wear comfortable, appropriate clothing. Tight clothes make you feel uneasy, especially in the torso. Loose and comfortable clothes can make you relax and feel free when you walk.

# References

1. Judith A. Chase, "Outpatient Management of Lower Back Pain," *Orthopaedic Nursing* 11, no. 1 (January/February 1992).
2. David Imrie, *The Back Power Program* (New York: Wiley, 1990).
3. John Frymoyer, "Back Pain and Sciatica," *New England Journal of Medicine* 318, no. 5 (1988): 291–300.
4. Evelyn Zamula, "Back Talk: Advice for Suffering Spines," *FDA Consumer*, April 1989.
5. Oliver Fultz, "Backaches," *American Health*, November 1991.
6. C. Lee., "Office Management of Lower Back Pain," *Orthopedic Clinics of North America* 19, no. 4 (1988): 797–804.
7. A. Fast, "Low Back Disorders: Conservative Management," *Archives of Physical Medicine and Rehabilitation* 69, no. 10 (1988): 880–891.
8. C. Evans, J. Gilbert, W. Taylor, et al., "A Randomized Controlled Trial of Flexion Exercises, Education, and Bed Rest for Patients with Acute Lower Back Pain," *Physiotherapy Canada* 39, no. 2 (1987): 96–101.
9. R. Million, W. Hall, K. Nilsen, et al., "Assessment of the Progress of the Back-Pain Patient," *Spine*, 7, no. 3 (1987): 204–212.
10. R. Deyo, "Conservative Therapy for Lower Back Pain," *Journal of American Medical Association* 250, no. 8 (1983): 1057–1062.
11. J. Sikorski, "A Rationalized Approach to Physiotherapy for the Back Pain," *Spine* 10, no. 6 (1985).
12. Alvin Nagelberg and Joanne Swanson, "Studies Find Adverse Effects of Cigarette Smoking," *P. M. Release*, February 18, 1993, papers 8 and 520.

# CHAPTER 5

# Qigong for Back Pain

## 5-1. Introduction

Before proceeding any further, we would first like to discuss the attitude you must have in your practice. Quite frequently, people who are ill are reluctant to get involved in the healing process. This is especially true for back pain patients. Both Western and traditional Chinese physicians have had difficulty persuading people to get involved in regular exercise or qigong. The main reason for this reluctance is that the patients are afraid of pain and therefore believe that these kinds of exercise are harmful. In order to conquer this obstacle to your healing, you must understand the theory of healing and the reason for practicing. Only then will you have the confidence necessary for continued practice. Remember, a physician may have an excellent prescription for your illness, but if you don't take the medicine, it won't do you any good.

Another factor that has caused the failure of many a potential cure is giving up too soon. Because the healing process is very slow, it is very easy to become impatient or to think the process is not working. Very often in life, we will know exactly what it is that we need to do, but because we are controlled by the emotional parts of our minds, we end up either not doing what we need to or not doing it right. Either way, our efforts have all been in vain.

It seems that most of the time our "emotional mind" (xin) and "wisdom mind" (yi) are in opposition. In China there is a proverb: "You are your own biggest enemy." This means that your emotional mind often wants to go in the opposite direction from what your wisdom mind knows is best. If your wisdom mind is able to conquer and govern your emotional mind, then there is nothing that can stop you from doing anything you want. Usually, however, your emotional mind makes you lazy, causes you to feel embarrassment, and destroys your willpower and perseverance. We always know that our clear-headed wisdom mind understands what needs to be done, but too often, we surrender to our emotional mind and become a slave of our emotions. When this happens, we usually feel guilty deep down in our hearts, and we try to find a good excuse so that we won't have to feel so guilty.

The first step when you decide to practice qigong is to strengthen your wisdom mind and use it to govern your emotional mind. Only then will you have enough patience and perseverance to keep practicing. You can see that the first key to successful training is not the techniques themselves but rather your self-control. I sincerely believe that as long as you have strong will, patience, and perseverance, there is nothing that can't be accomplished.

Forming the habit of practicing on a regular basis actually represents changing your lifestyle. Regulating your life through qigong can not only cure your back pain and restrengthen your spine, but it can also keep you healthy and make both your mental and physical lives much happier.

In this chapter, we will introduce some qigong practices that have proven to have great success in curing and preventing back pain. Although there are four fields of Chinese treatment for back pain, as mentioned earlier, because I am not qualified or experienced in the area of herbal and acupuncture treatments, I will focus on only qigong exercise. Still, I would like to remind you that among the four Chinese treatment methods, even though the other methods can alleviate pain, only qigong exercise is able to restrengthen and rebuild the strong root of the healthy spine.

In the next section, we will discuss a few important training procedures and keys. Without understanding these essential keys to training, the effectiveness of your practice will be shallow. In chapter 6, qigong exercises for back pain will be introduced for the reconditioning of your back. If you have a hard time learning these movements, you may also obtain a video that will demonstrate the movements clearly.

# 5-2. Important Training Keys

In this section, we will first address the five important regulating procedures for successful qigong training. Understanding these five factors will lead you to a deep level of practice. Naturally, the results will also be much greater.

After this, we will summarize some important keys for qigong practice. If you can comprehend these keys, you will have grasped the secret of qigong practice.

## Five Regulatings (Wu Tiao)

### 1. Regulating the Body

Before you start your qigong exercises, you should first calm down your mind and use this calm mind to bring your body into a calm and relaxed state. Naturally, you should always be concerned with your mental and physical centers. Only then will you be able to find your balance. When you have both mental and physical relaxation, centering and balance, you will be both natural and comfortable. This is the key to regulating your body.

When you relax, you should learn to relax deeply into your internal organs and especially the muscles that enclose the organs. In addition, you must also place your mind on the joints that are giving you trouble. The more you can bring your mind deep into the joint and relax it, the more qi will circulate smoothly and freely to repair the damage.

## 2. Regulating the Breathing

As mentioned before, breathing is the central strategy in qigong practice. According to qigong theory, when you inhale, you lead qi inward, and when you exhale, you lead qi outward. This is our natural process and we instinctually make use of it. For example, when you feel cold in the wintertime, in order to keep from losing qi out of your body, you naturally inhale more than you exhale to lead the qi inward, which also closes the pores in the skin. However, in the summertime when you are too hot, you naturally exhale more than you inhale in order to lead qi out of your body. When you do this, you start to sweat, and the pores open.

In qigong practice, generally, you want to lead the qi to the internal organs and bone marrow, so you must learn how to use inhalation to lead the qi inward. In addition, you would also like to lead the qi outward to the skin surface and beyond to strengthen your guardian qi (wei qi). Sometimes called protective qi, your guardian qi is a protective shield against negative qi influences around you.

When you use qigong to cure your back pain, you must learn how to inhale and exhale deeply and calmly so that you can lead the qi deep into the joints and also outward to dissipate the excess or stagnant qi that has accumulated in the joints. Therefore, in addition to relaxing when you practice, you should always remember to inhale and exhale deeply. When you inhale, place your mind deep in the joint, and when you exhale, lead the qi to the surface of the skin.

There are more than ten different methods of breathing in Chinese qigong practice. However, there are only two that are commonly used in our daily life. One is called abdominal breathing, or Buddhist breathing, and the other is called reverse abdominal breathing, or Daoist breathing. A key component, unique to Eastern training, is the use of the huiyin cavity (perineum). Traditionally, a master would not reveal this secret of huiyin control to any student until he was completely trusted by the master. It is shared with you in hopes that the deeper training be sustained.

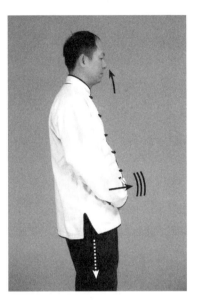

■ In normal abdominal breathing, when you inhale, gently push out your abdomen.

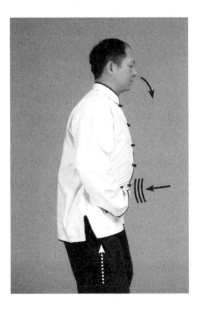

■ When you exhale, withdraw the abdomen.

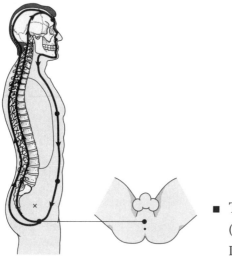

- The Huiyin Cavity (Co-1)
  (© LifeArt Collection of
  Images, Columbus, OH)

In order to fill up the qi to an abundant level in the lower abdominal area, when you inhale, you should also gently push your

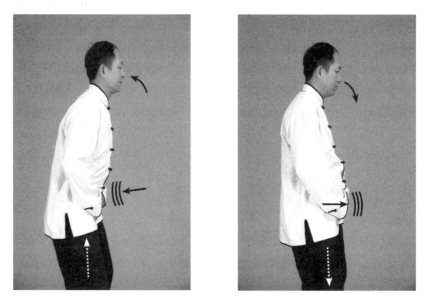

- In reverse abdominal breathing, when you inhale, the abdomen is gently pulled inward, and when you exhale, the abdomen is gently pushed outward.

huiyin (Co-1) cavity (or anus) out, and when you exhale, you hold it up gently. Remember, you should not tense this area during either inhalation or exhalation unless you are doing some special training such as hard qigong. Tension in this area can make the qi circulation stagnant.

Again, the coordination of the huiyin (Co-1) cavity (or anus) is very important. The huiyin ("meeting yin") cavity is a major gate that regulates the four yin vessels and, therefore, controls the qi status of the body.

When you practice reverse abdominal breathing, as you inhale, you should gently pull your huiyin (Co-1) cavity (or anus) up, and as you exhale, you should gently push it out. Again, you should not tense this area during either inhalation or exhalation unless you are doing some special training such as hard qigong.

Often, a qigong beginner will mistakenly believe that reverse abdominal breathing is not natural. On the contrary, reverse abdominal breathing is one of our normal breathing habits. Ordinarily, if your emotions are not disturbed or you do not have any intention to energize your muscular power to a higher level, you use normal breathing. However, when your emotional mind is disturbed, you may change your breathing into reverse breathing without realizing it. For example, when you are happy and laugh, you exhale while making the sound of "ha" and your abdominal area pushes out. When you are sad and cry, you inhale while making the sound of "hen" and your abdomen is withdrawn. Also, when you are scared, you inhale while holding your abdomen inward.

As mentioned previously, another occasion in which you use reverse breathing is when you have an intention to energize your muscular power to a higher, more powerful and spiritual state. For example, if you are pushing a car or lifting a heavy weight, you will use reverse breathing. In order to manifest your power to a higher level in martial arts, you must train your reverse breathing technique to be more efficient. This is the secret of jin and the way of Dao.

Often, a qigong or martial arts beginner encounters the problem of tightness in the abdominal area. The reason for this is that in reverse breathing, when you inhale, the diaphragm is pulling downward while the abdominal area is withdrawing. This can generate tension in the stomach area. To reduce this problem, you must start on a small scale with reverse breathing, and only after you can control the muscles in the abdominal area efficiently, gradually relax the area and eliminate the problem. Naturally, this will take time.

## 3. Regulating the Mind

As we noted earlier, in qigong, the mind is considered the general who directs the battle against sickness. After all, it is your mind that manages all of your thinking and activity. Therefore, a clear, calm mind is very important so that you can judge clearly and accurately. In addition, your mind must also be concentrated. Your mind can generate an electromotive force (or "voltage difference"), which causes your qi to circulate. The more you concentrate, the stronger you can lead the qi.

When you have a calm and concentrated mind, you can feel and sense the problem correctly. Therefore, when you practice qigong for your back pain, you must learn how to bring your mind inward so that you can understand the situation, and you must use your concentrated mind to lead the qi.

In practice, when you regulate your mind, you must, at the same time, coordinate with your breathing. If your breathing is deep and calm, your mind can be led to a profound meditative state. Moreover, normally when you inhale longer than you exhale, you can calm down easily. The other side of the token is that if you exhale longer than you inhale, you will be excited and lead the mind outside of your body.

Therefore, in order to lead your mind into your body, you must calm down and inhale deeply and slenderly, while physically becoming extremely relaxed. Once you can calm down your mind, you should then bring it to your third eye (or upper dan tian), located on your forehead. From both Chinese and ancient Western spiritual experience, it is recognized that paying attention to this spot is a way to lead your mind from outside of your body to an inner awareness. The reason for this, it is believed, is that our conscious mind (i.e., spirit) resides here.

If you practice correctly, you will soon feel that as you breathe, this place is harmonizing with your breathing. You will feel warmth and a very little pressure on this spot. If you can pay attention to this place for a few minutes, you will gradually lead your mind to an awareness of your inner feelings.

Next, move your mind from your third eye to your sternum. This area is considered to be the middle dan tian, which accumulates the fire qi. In Chinese qigong, it is believed that the fire qi at the middle dan tian will make you excited and emotional. Therefore, in order to lead your mind to a deeper and calmer meditative state, you must learn how to calm the fire at the middle dan tian. Therefore, you inhale deeply and use your mind to lead the qi from the middle dan tian to the lungs, and when you exhale, simply relax your lungs. The lungs are considered to be metal in Chinese five element medical philosophy. Metal is able to lead the heat away and therefore cool the fire. That is why whenever we are excited, if we inhale deeply and then relax, we can calm down easily. Through this breathing practice, you will have cooled off your excited energy, which is the key trick to leading your mind to the second phase of deep meditation.

Finally, lead your mind to your lower dan tian and keep it there for a while with the coordination of deep breathing. This will help you calm down to the deepest possible meditative state. When you are in this state, your mind will be very clear and feel what is happening in your body. If you are interested in knowing more about how to use your mind to lead both your mental and physical bodies into a deeply relaxed and meditative state, you may refer to the book *The Essence of Shaolin White Crane*, published by YMAA.

## 4. Regulating the Qi

Once you have regulated your body, breathing, and mind, you will already be in a good condition to start regulating your qi and can lead your qi anywhere in your body to make repairs.

If you have an injury or some damage that you need to repair, you should first inhale and use your mind to lead the qi to the deep place of the area, then exhale and again use your mind to lead the qi away from the place. If you do this correctly, you will soon feel this place grow warm with a sensational feeling that coordinates with your breathing.

## 5. Regulating the Spirit

The final key to qigong is raising your spirit of vitality. Good morale or fighting spirit is necessary to win the fight against illness. When your spirit is high, your willpower is strong, your mind is firm, and your patience can last long. In addition, when your spirit is high, your emotions are under control, and your wisdom mind can be calm and lead the qi to circulate in the body more efficiently. This will significantly reduce the time for healing.

You should now have a clear idea of how to practice most efficiently. During the course of your practice you should frequently remind yourself of these key requirements. If you would like to learn more about these keys to qigong practice, you may refer to the book *The Root of Chinese Qigong* (YMAA, 1997).

# Important Keys to Practice

Here we will list a few important keys to practice. These keys originated from many ancient qigong masters after a lifetime of experience. Naturally, most of these keys are closely related or linked with the five regulatings discussed above.

**Balance of Body and Heart (Emotional Mind) (Shen Xin Ping Heng).** In Chinese qigong, a human has two bodies: the physical body and the qi (energy) body. When these two bodies are harmonized and united with each other, you will be healthy and the spirit can be raised. In order to reach this goal, you must first regulate your mind. That means you should learn how to use your wisdom mind (yi) to govern your emotional mind (xin). Only then can your mind be calm and remain emotionally neutral. Under these conditions, your judgment can be accurate. When you use this clear mind to balance your physical and qi body's conditions, they can work together and coordinate with each other harmoniously.

**Unification of Internal and External (Nei Wai He Yi).** When you use a clear and wise mind to make good judgments, your physical body (external), mind (internal), and qi (internal) will all work together as one unit. However, even this does not mean that they can harmonize with one another. Only when they are harmonized can mutual coordination be achieved and the spirit of life be heightened. When you reach this stage, it is called "nei wai xie he," which means "mutual harmonization of internal and external."

In order to reach this level, you must first learn how to regulate your mind and bring it into the internal feeling of your body. If your mind cannot be restrained internally, you will not be able to feel any physical problem or qi imbalance in your body. This kind of practice is called "nei shi fan ting," which means "to see internally and to listen inwardly." Because it will take a great deal of patience and time to train this, it is also called "nei shi gongfu," which means "gongfu of internal vision."

If we apply the above concepts to our qigong healing for back pain, we must first educate our mind to understand the structure of our physical body, especially in the lower back area. From this understanding, we can comprehend the problem and know the situation clearly. Moreover, our mind must also be able to feel the qi imbalance in our body. Once your mind knows both the physical body (yang) and the qi body (yin) clearly, then you can adopt the treatments wisely to solve any problem.

To make the healing most effective, you should do more than just learn the techniques. More important is that through your mind's coordination, you make your physical body and qi body harmonize with each other smoothly. When this happens, the healing process will be fast and effective.

In order to harmonize the external with the internal, you must first learn how to regulate your body and perform the movements smoothly. When it is necessary to be relaxed, you are relaxed, and when it is necessary to be tensed, there is adequate tension. If you can do this, then you can adjust the depth of healing according to your inner feeling and understanding.

In addition, you must also learn how to use your mind to govern your breathing and coordinate with your external physical movements. Once you have reached a high level of coordination and harmonization of your mind, physical body, breathing, and qi body, you will have accomplished 90 percent of healing.

**Mutual Dependence of Heart (Mind) and Breathing (Xin Xi Xiang Yi).** In order to reach the final harmonization of the physical body and the qi body, your mind must always pay attention to your breathing. Breathing is considered to be the strategy. When the strategy is correct, the action can be effective, and the result can be fruitful. If your mind and breathing are coordinating with each other smoothly, the qi can be led effectively, naturally, and smoothly.

**Use the Yi (Wisdom Mind) to Lead the Qi (Yi Yi Yin Qi).**
Once you have good coordination of your physical body and qi body, then you learn how to use your mind to lead the qi. Naturally, the first step is learning how to keep your mind at the lower dan tian (bioelectric battery) located at your physical center. When your mind is able to stay in this center anytime you want, then physically you have a balance of the top and bottom, left and right, and front and rear. Not only that, the distribution of qi will also be balanced. When you are in this centered state, you are relaxed and mentally neutral. This practice is called "yi shou dan tian," which means "(wisdom) mind is kept at dan tian." This is the process of learning how to preserve the qi and store it in the human battery without wasting it. Theoretically speaking, the more you learn how to conserve your qi, the longer your vital force can last.

The next step is learning how to use the mind to lead the qi to the physically damaged place for repair. It is believed in Chinese medicine that as long as we provide the right condition for the cells to multiply, any physical damage in our body can be repaired. The first requirement is to provide plenty of qi. Without this qi, the repair will be slow or nonexistent.

The trick to using the mind to lead the qi is in the spirit (shen). It is known in Chinese qigong society that when the spirit is high, the qi can be led efficiently. Spirit is like the morale of a soldier. When morale is high, the soldier's fighting capability and potential is high. That is why it is said, "yi shen yu qi," which means, "use the shen to govern the qi." It is also said, "Your yi is on the spirit of vitality, not on your qi. (If) your yi in on your qi, (circulation of qi) will be stagnant."

The way of building up your spirit is to first establish your positive attitude. That means confidence and a strong will. Without these two factors, you will not be able to conquer sickness.

# 5-3. Qigong Exercises for Back Pain

Out of all the Chinese martial qigong developed in the last fifteen hundred years, there are only a few styles that pay attention to the torso's strength, especially the spine. These styles are White Crane, Snake, Dragon, and taijiquan. The reason for this is simply that these styles are classified as either soft or soft-hard styles of martial arts in China. In order to manifest martial power softly and strongly, the condition of the spine is critical. Without the strong foundation of the torso, not only will power not be manifested forcefully, but there may also be spinal injury.

Since ancient times, these few styles have been recognized as the best qigong exercises for spinal conditioning. Many traditional Chinese physicians have since adopted these qigong practices as a way of spinal rehabilitation for those patients with spine problems.

At this point, you may be curious as to why so many qigong healing exercises were developed in Chinese martial arts society, especially in the Buddhist and Daoist martial arts monasteries. If we examine Chinese martial arts history, we can see that often Chinese martial artists were training in the deep mountains with masters. Because there was usually no doctor in the deep mountains, whenever there was an injury, the martial artists needed to take care of it by themselves. After a few thousand years of self-healing practice, Chinese martial artists became experts in treating injury and have been recognized as one of the highest authorities on many kinds of injury treatments in Chinese medical society. The common treatments are massage, herbs, and qigong exercises.

The following qigong exercises are mainly from White Crane and taijiquan martial arts. The reason for this is simply that these are the two styles with which I am most familiar. It is well known that the key to becoming an expert is to practice continuously, to ponder, and to accumulate experience. Experience is the best teacher. As long as you remain humble, ponder, and combine theory and practice, you will soon become an expert in dealing with spinal problems. If you are interested in knowing more about White Crane and taiji qigong, please refer to the books *The Essence of Shaolin White Crane* and *The Essence of Taiji Qigong*, published by YMAA.

# CHAPTER 6

# Qigong Exercises

EXTERNAL QIGONG IS ALSO called dan (external elixir) qigong, because it emphasizes external physical movements and uses the mind to lead the qi to the extremities or local areas of the body either for healing or physical strengthening. External qigong can be classified as soft, soft-hard, and hard. In the soft category, the muscles and tendons are relaxed to a deep level while moving the joints. The main purpose of this soft external qigong is that through repeating the movements, the ligaments are exercised and the blood circulation in the deep places of the joints is improved.

Soft-hard external qigong moves the joints softly while twisting the joints or slightly tensing the tendons in the joint areas. The main purpose of this qigong is to strengthen the structure of the joints, such as ligaments and tendons. Again, through repeating the movements, the joints are conditioned gradually. Any injury in the joints can be repaired due to the enhanced qi and blood circulation.

Finally, hard external qigong is used to build up the strength and endurance of the muscles and tendons. Normally, only the physical tension can be seen externally. This qigong is not too much different from that practiced in the lifting of weights. The only difference is the use of the mind. In qigong, the mind is used to lead the qi to the muscular body first before it is tensed. From this mind and body coordination, the efficiency and effectiveness of exercises can be enhanced to a higher level. As mentioned earlier, this is called the unification of the internal and external.

Past experience teaches that in order to improve the qi and blood circulation in the deep places of the joints, we must first loosen up the joints. After loosening up the joints, a gentle and firm stretching should follow in order to open up the joints, especially if there is any injury or pain in them. Then, correct joint movements should be done repeatedly until the joints are warm. Finally, joint-loosening exercises should be used to lead the qi away from the joints.

Next, we will introduce qigong exercises for back pain. Before you start, you should recognize an important fact. After your exercise, you may find that your back or torso muscles are more sore and painful than before. This is quite normal. There are two reasons for this. First, you are exercising muscles and tendons that you seldom exercised before. Their condition is weak. Therefore, you should start the following exercises with only a few repetitions at first. Only if you feel stronger should you increase the number of repetitions. That means you are conditioning your physical body from weak to strong.

Second, after you exercise, the circulation of the qi and blood will be enhanced. This will enliven your nervous system at the local area and make it more sensitive. When this happens, you will experience soreness. You should not be discouraged by this. Treat it as a challenge. Remember, the more you move, the better your physical condition will become. However, should you feel sharp pain, burning, tingling, or a pain that radiates down into your legs, you should again reduce the number of repetitions and consult with your doctor.

# 6-1. Loosening Up the Lower Back

The main goal is to loosen up any tightness in the waist area caused from back pain. When you are doing the loosening-up exercises, you should breath naturally. Do not hold your breath. Holding your breath will make your muscles tense.

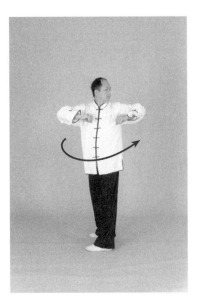

■ Place both arms right in front of your chest with palms facing downward. Then, turn your body from side to side gently. This will loosen up the torso muscles and excite them gradually. Repeat about six times to each side.

■ Continue to keep both your arms right in front of your chest. Loosen up your torso by moving your hips forward to generate an upward wave motion while circling both your arms upward, forward, and then downward in a continuous motion. The intention of this movement is to move the torso gently to loosen up the muscles.

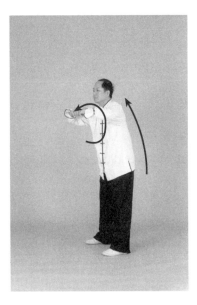

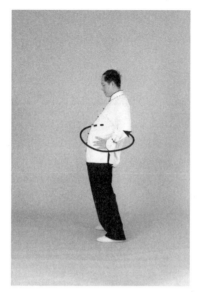

- Place your hands on your waist and then circle your waist horizontally. Circle in one direction and then the other, a few times in each direction. If you experience any pain, make the circles smaller. However, if you feel comfortable and there is not too much pain, you may increase the size of the circular motion and also the number of circles. This will loosen up the lower back area and the hip joints. Only you can decide how big the circle should be.

# 6-2. Stretching

After you have loosened up your waist area, you should start to stretch your torso. If you stretch your torso correctly, you will stimulate the cells into an excited state, and this will improve qi and blood circulation. This is the key to maintaining the health of the physical body. However, when you stretch, you should treat your muscles, tendons, and ligaments like a rubber band. Stretch gently and gradually. If you stretch the rubber band too much and too fast, it will break. For muscles, tendons, and ligaments, that means the tearing off of fibers. However, if you understretch, it will not be effective. A good stretch should feel comfortable and stimulating.

When you practice the stretching, do not hold your breath. If you hold your breath, your body will be tense. How far you should stretch depends on your feeling. If you feel pain, producing both physical tension and mental disturbance, then you may have pushed too far. Proceed cautiously and gently, and push a little bit farther each time. You are looking for progress but without feeling uncomfortable pain.

# Stretching the Torso (Shuang Shou Tuo Tian)

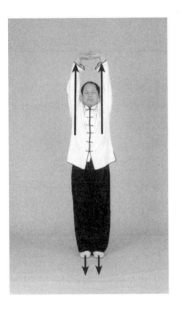

■ First, interlock your fingers. As you lift your interlocked hands up over your head, rotate your hands so the palms face upward. Imagine that you are pushing upward with your hands and pushing downward with your feet. Do not tense your muscles, because this will constrict your body and prevent you from stretching. If you do this stretch correctly, you will feel the muscles in your waist area tensing slightly because they are being pulled simultaneously from the top and the bottom. Next, use your mind to relax and stretch out a little bit more. Remember to keep your palms turned directly upward; don't allow them to roll toward the front. Also, be careful. Do not thrust out the lower ribs. Keep your pelvis level.

- After you have stretched for about ten seconds, twist your upper body to one side to twist the trunk muscles. Stay twisted to the side for three to five seconds, then turn your body to face forward. Turn to the other side. Stay twisted to this side for three to five seconds, then return to face forward. Repeat the upper-body twisting three times. Come back to the center.

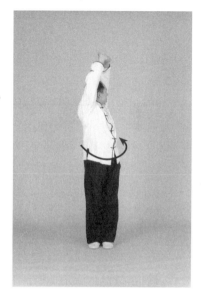

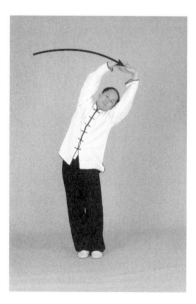

- Next, tilt your upper body to the side and stay there for about three to five seconds, then tilt to the other side. Repeat three times, maintaining the feeling of stretching upward throughout the entire process.

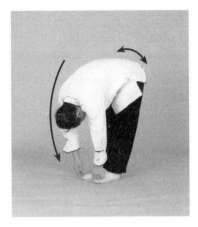

- Next, bend forward gently and use your pelvis to wave the hips from side to side to loosen up the lower spine. Bring your hips back to center and stay there for ten seconds.

- Finally, if possible, squat down with your feet flat on the ground to stretch your ankles.

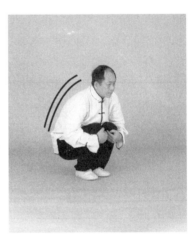

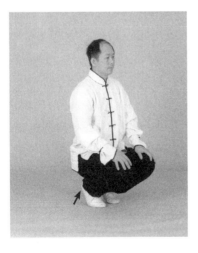

- Then lift your heels up to stretch the toes.

Repeat the entire process three times. After you finish, the inside of your body should feel very comfortable and warm.

If you are already in good health, you can do the following variation, which provides a more aggressive stretch to reach the ligaments.

- Clasp your fingers and raise your hands over your head, rotating the hand so the palms face the ceiling. When your arms are up above your head, keep the torso stretched while circling your waist area. Try six circulations to each side at the beginning. Remember, too much exercise may cause injury and too little will not be effective. You are the one who should make the judgment.

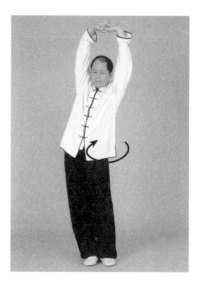

## Stretching and Loosening Up the Neck

After you have stretched your torso, you should next stretch your neck. The neck is the junction of the blood-and-qi-exchanging path between the head and the body. Whenever the neck is stiffened or the spine in the neck is injured, this blood-and-qi exchange will be stagnant. Consequently, your brain will not have proper nourishment. In addition, the muscles in the neck extend downward to the chest and the back. Whenever the back is tense, the neck is also stiff and vice versa. Therefore, in order to maintain your health and relieve back tension, you must also learn the correct manner of loosening up the neck, including the muscles, tendons, and ligaments.

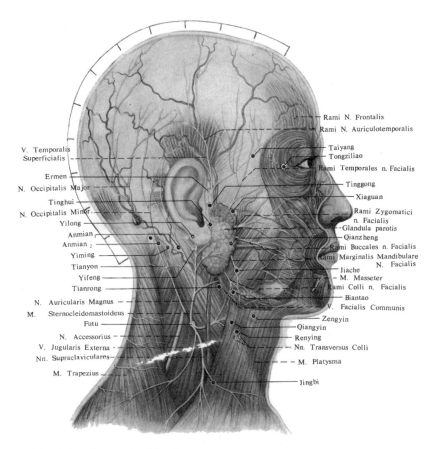

■ The Muscles in the Neck

First, stretch the muscles and tendons around the neck and gradually reach to the ligaments, which are hidden deeply between the joints. To stretch the neck muscles and tendons, you should focus on the four biggest muscles and tendons located on the front and the back side of your neck.

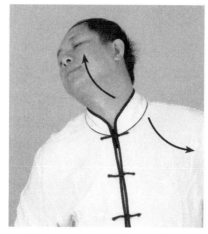

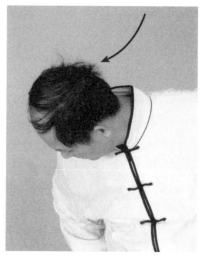

- When you stretch your front neck muscles and tendons, you may turn your head backward diagonally while pressing your shoulder backward. Start the stretching gently for twenty seconds.

- Then shift the stretching to the rear neck muscles and tendons. When you stretch your rear neck muscles and tendons, simply press your head downward and toward the side. Stretch for twenty seconds.

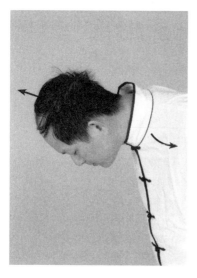

After you have gone through the four sets of muscles and tendons, repeat from the beginning for another twenty seconds each. You should stretch each muscle and tendon group at least three times. This will provide good stimulation to the muscles and tendons through stretching.

After you have stretched the four neck muscle and tendon groups, extend your head forward

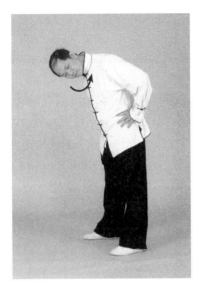

- Then turn your head to your left slowly and then to your right slowly. This will help you stretch and loosen up the ligaments in the neck. Repeat the turning two more times to each side.

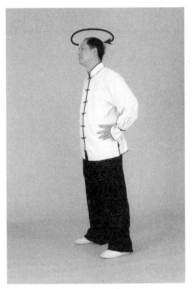

- Finally, gently circle your head, on a small scale, in one direction about ten times and then the other direction for another ten times. You should not circle your neck to its extreme range of motion because this may damage your cartilage and neck joints. This is a common cause of arthritis in the lower neck area in later life.

with the four muscle and tendon groups evenly stretched. To make the stretching more efficient, you may gently push both of your shoulders backward. The goal is to stretch the ligaments instead of the muscles and tendons. Stay in this stretching position for twenty seconds.

# 6-3. Spine Qigong

Next, we will introduce two qigong exercise sets that can be used to heal and rebuild the strength of the back. The first is a set of moving soft and soft-hard qigong developed from White Crane and taijiquan martial styles. It is well known that soft and soft-hard qigong can be used to improve the qi and blood circulation and also to rebuild the strength of the ligaments, tendons, and muscles in the back. Therefore, these exercises can be used effectively and efficiently for healing if you have already had a back pain problem. In fact, these soft and soft-hard qigong sets are recommended for those who have already had some back pain problems. Generally, if you do these exercises twice per day, you should see some significant improvement in three months and nearly complete healing in six months. Qigong is not a drug but an exercise to rebuild the strength of your physical body. It takes both time and patience.

The first set is designed for those who have already experienced significant pain and cannot move their spine comfortably while standing.

The second set is a stationary soft-hard qigong that was developed in the Shaolin Temple. The training aims for the reconditioning and rebuilding of the strength and endurance of the muscles and tendons. Once your body has good support from strong torso muscles and tendons, the pressure on the vertebrae joints will be significantly reduced. It is commonly known that when the torso muscles and tendons are weak due to aging or lack of exercise, the pressure on the vertebrae joints will be increased.

From this, you can see that when you do moving soft and soft-hard spinal qigong, the exercises can reach deeply, and healing will be more internal. Once you have cured the problem, you must build up a firm and strong physical torso.

# Moving Soft and Soft-Hard Qigong

The torso is supported by the spine and the trunk muscles. Once you have stretched your trunk muscles, you can loosen up the torso. This also moves around the muscles inside your body, which moves and relaxes your internal organs. This, in turn, makes it possible for the qi to circulate smoothly inside your body.

Once you have mastered all of the movements, you should learn to bring your mind into a deeper meditative state, which allows you to feel and sense the deeper places in your body. Then, through the coordination of the mind, the breathing, and the physical movements, lead the qi to the injured place for healing, and lead the accumulated stagnant qi away from the injured area. We have explained the theory of all of these internal practices in the earlier sections. To make the healing more effective, you need the "unification and harmonization of the internal and external."

In this subsection, I would like first to introduce the spine exercises from a standing position. Then, I will present some new concepts for supine spinal exercises for those who cannot stand up and move the spine easily.

### Standing Spine Sigh Movement (Jizhui Tan Xi)

Spine sigh movement is very important to the back pain patient. This movement imitates the spine's natural action when you make a sigh. Normally, when you are making a deep sigh, you are sick, sad, or depressed. When this happens, your inhalation is longer than your exhalation, and the qi in your torso is more trapped inside, which can therefore cause your torso muscles and spine to become more tense. In addition, the qi stagnation can also occur in the internal organs and result in sickness. Under these circumstances, you will instinctively inhale deeply while thrusting your chest out and then push your pelvis out slightly to loosen the lower back.

Finally, release the carbon dioxide and continue pushing the lower back backward to relax it.

When you do this correctly, you will feel the relaxation so deeply in the spine that it reaches the ligaments of the vertebrae. Remember, whenever you experience lower back pain or tightness, the first step is to repeat this spine sigh movement to loosen up the lower back.

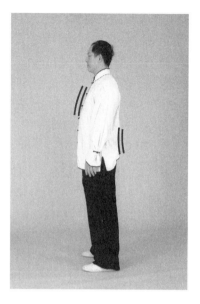

- Inhale deeply while thrusting your chest out.

- Then push your pelvis out slightly to loosen the lower back. Make the sound of "hen" as you exhale naturally while continuing to move your spine like a wave upward into the upper body. From these repeated sighing movements, the tension of the torso can be eased, and the internal organs can be more relaxed.

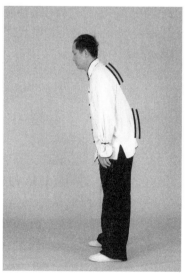

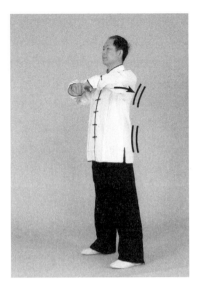
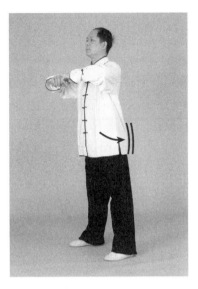

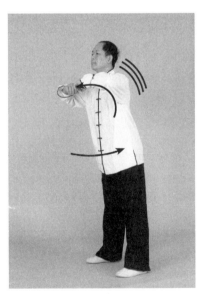

■ In order to become more familiar with this spine sigh movement, practice the next movement. Place both arms comfortably in front of your chest. When you inhale, thrust your chest out while straightening up your torso (tailbone pushed forward) and then continue your inhalation while pushing your pelvis backward and gradually holding in your chest.

When you push your pelvis backward, the mingmen (Gv-4) cavity on the back will be opened, and the qi in the front and the rear side of the torso will be balanced. Mingmen is translated as "life door" in Chinese medicine because it is understood that this is the gate that connects with the center of our life, the real lower dan tian (zhen xia dan tian). The mingmen cavity is located between the second and third lumbar vertebrae. To release tension in the lower

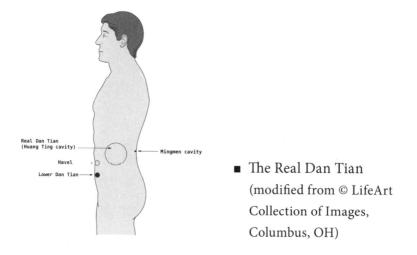

■ The Real Dan Tian (modified from © LifeArt Collection of Images, Columbus, OH)

back, the first task is to relax and open this gate by gently and slightly pushing the pelvis backward. If you have already experienced back pain, you must learn how to move your pelvis correctly to relax the lower back area.

## Standing Circle the Waist Horizontally (Pin Yuan Niu Yao)

This exercise helps you to regain conscious control of the muscles in your abdomen. The real lower dan tian is the main residence of your original qi (yuan qi). The qi in your real lower dan tian can be led easily only when your abdomen is loose and relaxed. These abdominal exercises are probably the most important of all the internal qigong practices.

- Squat down slightly. Without moving your thighs or upper body, use the waist muscles to move the abdomen around in a horizontal circle. You should pay attention to the circling of the lower back area. Circle in one direction about ten times and then in the other direction about ten times. If you hold one hand over your lower dan tian and the other on your sacrum, you may be able to focus your attention better on the area you want to control.

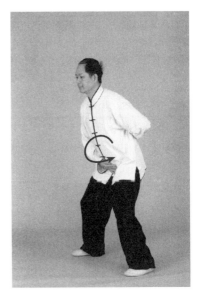

In the beginning, you may have difficulty making your body move the way you want. But if you keep practicing, you will quickly learn how to do it. Once you can do the movement comfortably, make the circles larger and larger. Naturally, this will cause the muscles to tense somewhat and inhibit the qi flow, but the more you practice, the sooner you will again be able to relax. After you have practiced for a while and can control your waist muscles easily, start making the circles smaller, and also start using your yi to lead the qi from the real lower dan tian to move in these circles. The final goal is to have only a slight physical movement but a strong movement of qi.

There are four major benefits to this abdominal exercise. First, when your real lower dan tian area is loose, the qi can flow in and out easily. This is especially important for health because the real lower dan tian is the main source of qi. Second, when the abdominal area is loose, the qi circulation in the large and small intestines will be smooth, and they can absorb nutrients and eliminate waste. If your body does not eliminate effectively, the absorption of nutrients will be hindered, and you may become sick. Third, when the abdominal area is loose, the qi in the kidneys will circulate smoothly, and the original essence (yuan jing) stored in the kidneys can be converted more efficiently into qi. In addition, when the kidney area is loosened, the kidney qi can bc led downward and upward to nourish the entire body. Fourth, these exercises eliminate qi stagnation in the lower back, healing and preventing lower back pain. Furthermore, this exercise can also help you rebuild the strength of the muscles in the waist area.

## Standing with Support Circle Waist

If you find that there is too much pain when you stand up to circle the lower back, you may use your hands to support part of the body's weight by leaning against a wall, chair, or table. The whole idea is to move the lower vertebrae and improve the qi and blood circulation there. Once you are stronger, you should practice standing and do more repetitions. How many circles you do in each practice depends on your condition. You should proceed cautiously and gradually.

- Place both hands on the back of a chair or table. Without moving your thighs or upper body, use the waist muscles to move the abdomen around in a horizontal circle. You should pay attention to the circling of the lower back area.

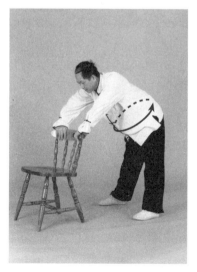

## Standing Waving the Spine and Massaging the Internal Organs (Ji Zhui Bo Dong, Nei Zang An Mo)

Beneath your diaphragm is your stomach. On its right is your liver and on its left is your spleen. Once you can comfortably do the movement in your lower abdomen, change the movement from horizontal to vertical, and extend it up to your diaphragm. Move your vertebrae joint by joint. What you are aiming for is the movement of the ligaments that connect the joints. The deep places of the joints must be moved in order to heal. The easiest way to loosen the area around the diaphragm is to use a wavelike motion between the perineum and the diaphragm.

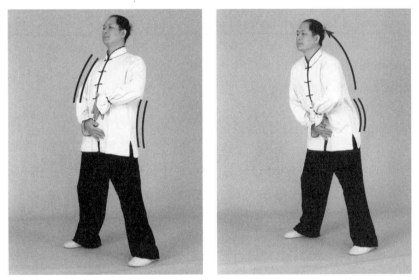

- You may find it helpful when you practice this to place one hand on your abdomen and your other hand above it with the thumb on the solar plexus.

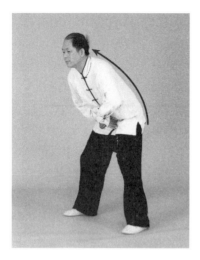

■ Use a forward and backward wavelike motion, flowing up to the diaphragm and down to the perineum and back. Practice ten times.

■ Continue the movement while turning your body slowly to one side and then to the other. This will slightly tense the muscles and tendons on one side and loosen them on the other, which will massage the internal organs. This will also gently and gradually stretch and condition the ligaments and rebuild the strength. Repeat ten times on each side.

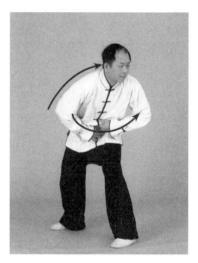

## Sitting Waving the Spine

If you have already experienced serious back pain, you may again use a chair or the wall to reduce the pressure on your vertebrae. You may practice this waving exercise while you are sitting either at the desk or while driving.

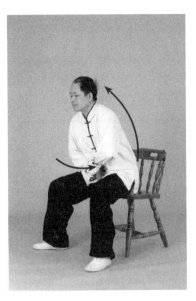

- Sit on the edge of a chair with your feet firmly on the ground. Use a forward and backward wavelike motion, flowing up to the diaphragm and down to the perineum and back. Practice ten times.

Whether standing or sitting, the most important part of this practice is to reach as deep as possible in the movements. In order to reach this goal, your mind must be able to reach deeply, and the movements of the muscles and tendons must be correct. Too tense is not good, and too relaxed will not serve any purpose.

## Standing Thrust the Chest and Arch the Chest (Tan Xiong Gong Bei)

After loosening up the center portion of your body, extend the movement up to your chest and upper spine. Remember the sigh movement? This exercise is actually a large-scale version of the same movement. The inhalation and exhalation should be as deep as possible, and the entire chest should be very loose. When you move your spine, you should be able to feel the vertebrae move section by section.

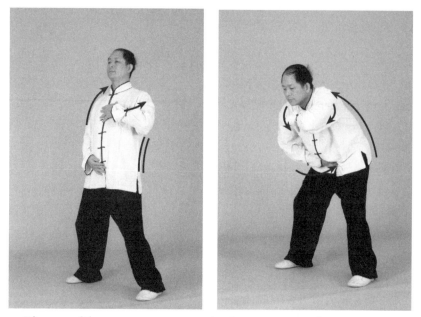

- The wavelike movement starts in the sacrum and moves up to the chest. You may find it easier to feel the movement if you hold one hand on your abdomen and the other lightly on your chest. You should also coordinate with the shoulders' movement. Inhale when you move your shoulders backward, and exhale when you move them forward.
- Repeat the motion ten times.

This exercise loosens up the chest and helps to regulate and improve the qi circulation in the lungs. Moreover, this kind of wavelike spine movement will not only improve the qi and blood circulation at the vertebrae joints for healing, but it will also gradually recondition your spine structure from weak to strong. Remember, spine movement is the key to maintaining spinal health. This is also the key to strengthening your immune system.

## Sitting Thrust the Chest and Arch the Chest

Again, you may practice this spine movement while sitting as well as standing.

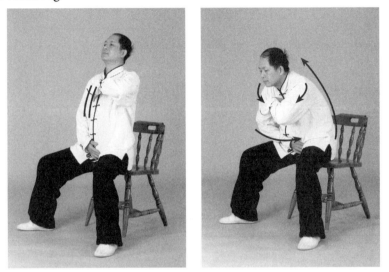

- Sit on the edge of a chair with your feet firmly on the ground. Generate the wave motion from the sacrum and move it upward while coordinating with your breathing.

Be aware of the stiffness of your spine whenever you sit for too long while either driving or working. Lift your arms up and stretch your torso first. Then perform the above spinal movements to exercise the spine and loosen it.

## Standing White Crane Waves Its Wings
## (Bai He Dou Chi)

Once you have completed the loosening up of the chest area and spine, extend the motion to your arms and fingers.

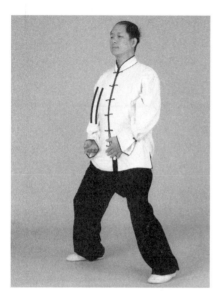

- Place both palms in front of your abdominal area, facing forward.

- Next, generate the wave motion from the legs or the waist and direct this power upward.

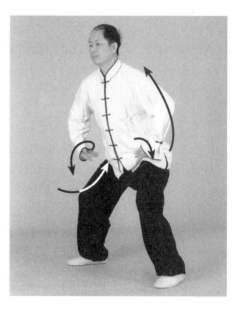

- The wave passes through the chest and shoulders and finally reaches the arms. Repeat at least ten times. Naturally, if you feel comfortable, you may practice more.

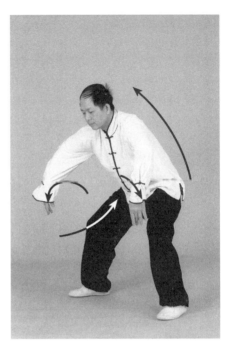

## Standing White Crane Waves Its Wing—Single Wing

Right after you have finished the above two-hands-waving exercises, you should then practice one-hand-waving exercises. The additional benefit you may obtain comes from twisting your joints from the ankles, hips, spine, and finally reaching to the fingertips. This will help to loosen and strengthen the joint areas.

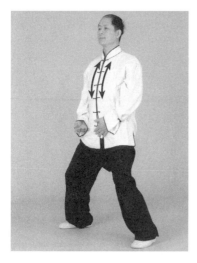

- When you practice with one arm, again you place both your palms right in front of your abdominal area with the right palm facing out and the left palm lightly touching the abdomen.

- Then, generate the twisting motion from the bottom of your feet upward through the knees and hips, through every section of the spine.

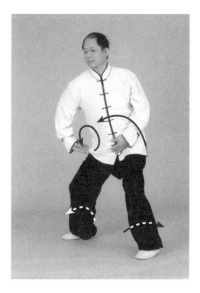

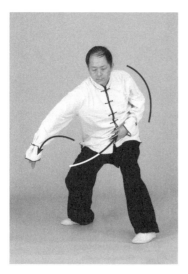

- Finally, allow it to pass through the shoulders and reach to the fingertips. Practice ten times for each arm.

Again, you may practice this qigong exercise while you are sitting.

## Sitting White Crane Waves Its Wings

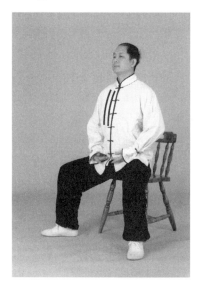

- Begin with both hands in front of your abdominal area.

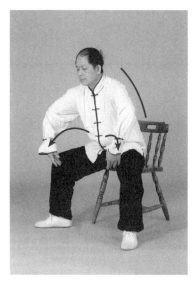

- The wave passes through the chest and shoulders and finally reaches the arms. Repeat at least ten times. Naturally, if you feel comfortable, you may practice more.

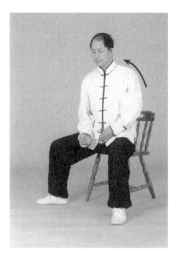

## Sitting White Crane Waves Its Wing—Single Wing

- Place both your palms right in front of your abdominal area with the right palm facing out and the left palm lightly touching the abdomen.

- Then, generate the twisting motion from the bottom of your feet, upward through the knees and hips, through every section of the spine. Finally, allow it to pass through the shoulders and reach to the fingertips. Practice ten times for each arm.

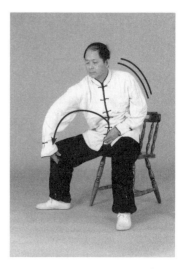

These exercises will loosen up every joint in your body from the waist to the fingers. Moreover, they lead the qi out from the central body to the limbs. If you are not leading the excess qi out, the body will become too yang and you may become tense again. The key to healing and relaxation is to lead the excess qi out of the body through the limbs. These movements have been found beneficial for healing chest problems such as asthma, chest cancer, lung problems, and heart problems.

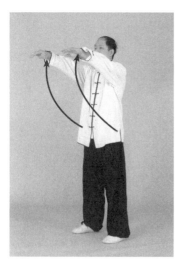

## Standing Recovery

After you have completed the above spine waving movements, continue to lead the qi out of your body through the limbs. The easiest way is to swing your arms forward and backward by imitating a natural human activity— walking.

- Swing your arms forward to the height of the shoulders.

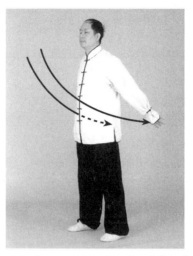

- Then, let your arms drop and swing back by themselves. Repeat about two hundred times.

You may swing your arms for five minutes to half an hour depending on your health. Swinging the arms is one of the easiest qigong practices, simple and easy for anyone.

- Next, continue your swinging while at the same time walking in place and bringing your knees as high as your hips. Every time you raise your knee, you gently push back your lower back. This will generate a comfortable forward and backward movement to exercise the lower back. Again, if it is comfortable, start with fifty steps, and when you feel stronger, increase the number of repetitions.

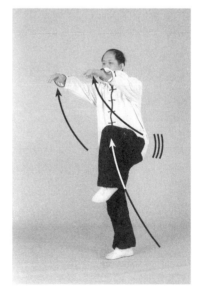

- Finally, you should lead the qi to the bottom of your feet. Continue your arm swinging. When your arms are lifting, raise your heels, and when your arms are down, make your heels touch the floor. Repeat about twenty to thirty times. If you start with more than thirty, you may experience cramping in your calf.

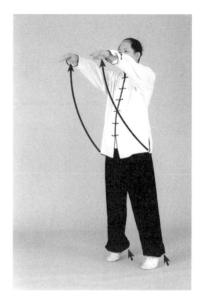

When you practice this exercise, you do not have to worry about your breathing. Simply breathe naturally and smoothly. You may even watch television while you are swinging your arms. This is why the recovery exercises can be called layperson's qigong. It is simple and easy, without too much training of concentrated mind and breathing.

# Exercises for Pain Relief

### On the Floor

If you have already had serious back problems, you may find the above exercises to be too strenuous. In this case, follow the exercises by using the floor, at least at first. After you feel stronger and more comfortable, you can practice normally.

The point of using the floor is to ease the pressure on your vertebrae by removing the upper body's weight.

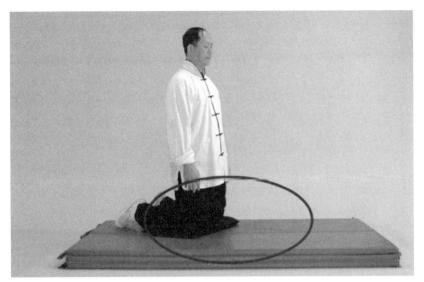

- The basic posture is kneeling down on the floor. If you can kneel down on some soft surface such as a pillow or a blanket, then the pressure on your knees will be minimized.

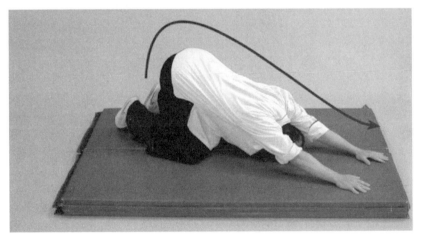

- Next, bend forward with both arms straightened forward so the torso can be gently stretched. If possible and comfortable, you should stretch your arms forward. This will help to open up the vertebrae joints significantly. You should stretch your torso straight forward for at least two minutes.

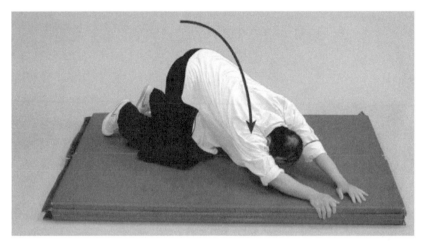

- Then, you move your arms to one side and stretch one side of your torso for another two minutes and then to the other side for two minutes.

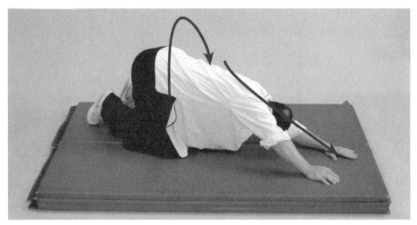

- Once you have finished stretching, move your arms back to the forward position. Next, move your waist area in circular motions. When you move your lower back backward, inhale, and when it moves downward, exhale. Begin with small circles and gradually increase the scale and number of circling, if and only if you feel comfortable. Circle to each direction about twenty times at first. When you feel comfortable, you may gradually increase the number of circles.

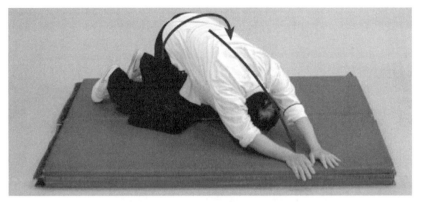

- Next, move your arms to one side and repeat the same exercises twenty times. Be sure to practice both sides.

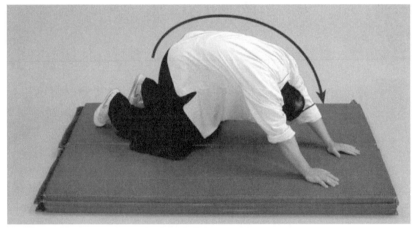

- Move your arms back to the forward position. Then, you should generate a wavelike movement, starting in the sacrum and moving up to the neck. Go easy and move slowly and gently, paying close attention. Remember, the deeper your concentration, the deeper you can feel. The deeper you can feel, the more you can regulate the problem. This is a meditative exercise. You must coordinate your breathing and your mind. When you initiate the movement, inhale, and when the wave is moving upward, exhale. Again, begin with smaller-scale motions, and only if you feel comfortable, increase their scale and numbers. Repeat this wavelike movement about twenty times.

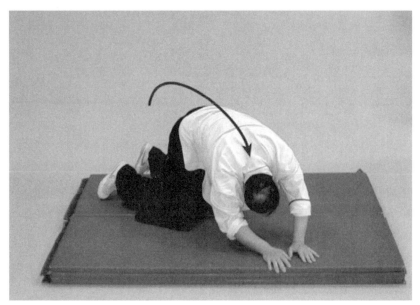

- Move your arms to one side and repeat the same wavelike motion twenty more times. Move your arms to the other side and repeat the wavelike motion twenty times.

After you have completed the exercises, you should lie comfortably for a few minutes before you stand up. This will allow the qi and blood to circulate while you relax. The exercises are most effective when practiced at least twice a day.

# Building Strength and Endurance

## Stationary Hard Qigong

As mentioned earlier, stationary hard qigong focuses on building the strength and endurance of the muscles and tendons. However, the training will contribute only slightly to the ligaments' reconditioning. The reason for this is simply that in order to build up the muscles and tendons and reach a healthy level, the muscles and tendons must be tensed up during the training. When this happens, the joints will be more tense and locked. This will therefore limit the mobility of the joint movements, and the ligaments will not be conditioned.

## Taiji Arching Arms (Taiji Gong Shou)

Taiji arching arms is a taiji training that specializes in conditioning the strength and endurance of the torso and spine, especially the lower back area. It is a standing-still meditation. This training is not as hard and tense as that of the Shaolin training called Iron Board Bridge, which will be introduced in the next section. Therefore, if you have treated your spine problem to a healthier level, you may want to strengthen your torso and increase its endurance gradually. This is the way to prevent back pain from happening again.

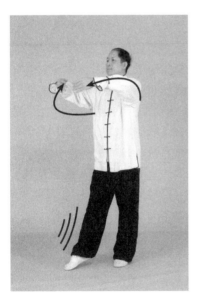

- Stand with one leg solidly on the ground while the other foot gently touches the floor with the toes. In addition, hold both your arms at shoulder height with your palms facing your chest.

When you do this, if your left foot is touching with the toes, your right side back muscles and tendons will be more tensed than the left side. You should stand in this position for three minutes at the beginning, and then switch your legs for another three minutes without moving your arms. This will condition the left side of back muscles and tendons. When you practice, breathe naturally and smoothly. If possible, keep your mind aware internally to feel the training, especially the torso's condition.

After you practice for a while and feel your torso getting stronger, you may increase the time for standing gradually. In taijiquan practice, often a practitioner will stand for fifteen to thirty minutes on each leg. Even though this training builds up strength and endurance slowly and gradually, there is no risk involved. It is recommended for people who have a weak torso and spine.

## Iron Board Bridge (Tie Ban Qiao)

Iron Board Bridge is well known in the external styles of Chinese martial arts. The main purpose of the training is to build up a stronger and more durable torso for power manifestation and also

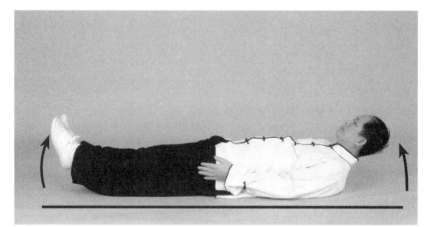

- When you begin this training, simply lie down with your face looking upward and lift your head and heels a couple of inches off the ground. The entire leg should be straight. The distance from your head to the ground and also from the heels to the ground should not be too high. If they are too high, pressure will build up in the lower spine and cause injury. A proper height for the lifting of the head and the heels can keep the rear side of the torso stretched and the front side properly tensed. Hold this position for thirty seconds to one minute.

to prevent injury to the spine. It is important to remember that if you have a weak back, you should consult with your doctor before you train Iron Board Bridge.

After you have trained for some time, if you feel comfortable, increase to two minutes and so on until you can hold it for three minutes. If you can reach this goal, you have built up a very good level of strength in your torso.

When you train, you should take your time. Do not hold your breath while training. Hasty training can only harm you. You should remember that your body must be conditioned slowly and gradually. If you have too much ego, once you have injured yourself, it will take a long time to heal, and once you have injured yourself, you will never be quite the same. The results of mistraining can be devastating. Remember, if you have a weak back, you must consult with your doctor before you train Iron Board Bridge.

The above qigong practices have been experienced for hundreds and some for a thousand years, and they have proven very effective and beneficial for spinal healing and rebuilding of strength. You should build up your confidence and proceed with healing and reconditioning slowly and gradually. Always pay attention to your body, feel it, and communicate with it. Moreover, you should also analyze and understand the conditions and the theory of the practice. Once you have built up a firm and solid theoretical and practical root, you may find other postures or movements that can help your healing and reconditioning to proceed faster and more suitably for you.

# Conclusion

I WOULD LIKE TO stress that this book is written based on my personal understanding and experience in treating lower back pain both from the Western and Chinese medical point of view. Moreover, because of the limitation of my personal knowledge and experience in acupuncture and herbal treatments for the same problem, I do not include these two methods of treatments in this book. I sincerely hope some qualified Chinese physician is able to write some books about these treatments to fill this void.

In addition, I would like to urge you to keep your mind open, study, and absorb other sources of information about back pain treatments. The more information you have, the more angles of seeing the same thing will be provided. This will help you analyze the problem more logically and wisely.

Finally, I would like to remind you that the most important part of the entire treatment is to rebuild the strength of your torso. This will take a great deal of patience and time. Therefore, the first and the most important task or challenge you must face is to establish your strong will and confidence. Without these factors, all of the methods you have read about in this book will be useless. You should not give up. Remember to also proceed cautiously with the treatment. Normally, it will take about three months of qigong exercise to see the primary result. Moreover, in order to maintain the health of your spine, you should not stop the qigong exercises even when the back pain is gone. Keep yourself in good shape and build up your firm and strong spirit. This is the way to prevent and fight against disease.

# Acknowledgments

The publisher wishes to thank Leslie Takao and Doran Hunter for editing, T. G. LaFredo for his supervision, and Tim Comrie for project management.

# Translation and Glossary of Chinese Terms

**an mo.** Literally, "press rub." Together they mean "massage."

**ba mai.** Referred to as the Eight Extraordinary vessels. These eight vessels are considered to be qi reservoirs, which regulate the qi status in the primary qi channels.

**Bai He.** Means "White Crane." One of the Chinese southern martial styles.

**baliao (B-31–34).** Eight cavities on the sacrum that belong to the bladder primary qi channels. Baliao includes shangliao, ciliao, zhongliao, and xialiao (four on each side of sacrum).

**changqiang (Gv-1).** Name of an acupuncture cavity that belongs to the governing vessel.

**chengfu (B-50).** An acupuncture cavity that belongs to the bladder primary qi channel.

**Cheng, Gin-Gsao.** Dr. Yang, Jwing-Ming's White Crane master.

**chi (qi).** The general definition of qi is: universal energy, including heat, light, and electromagnetic energy. A narrower definition of qi refers to the energy circulating in human or animal bodies. A current popular model is that the qi circulating in the human body is bioelectric in nature.

**chi kung (qigong).** Gong means gongfu (literally, "energy-time"). Therefore, qigong means study, research, and practices related to qi.

**chong mai.** Thrusting vessel. One of the eight extraordinary qi vessels.

**ciliao (B-32).** One of four cavities on each side of the sacrum that belongs to the bladder primary qi channel.

**dai mai.** Girdle (or belt) vessel. One of the eight qi vessels.

**dan tian.** Literally, "field of elixir." Locations in the body that are able to store and generate qi (elixir) in the body. The upper, middle, and lower dan tian are located, respectively, between the eyebrows, at the solar plexus, and a few inches below the navel.

**dan tian qi.** Usually, the qi converted from original essence and stored in the lower dan tian. This qi is considered "water qi" and is able to calm down the body. Also called xian tian qi (pre-heaven qi).

**Dao.** The "Way," by implication the "Natural Way."

**dian.** "To point" or "to press."

**dian qi.** Dian means "electricity" and so dian qi means "electrical energy" (electricity). In China, a word is often placed before "qi" to identify the different kinds of energy.

**dian xue.** Dian means "to point and exert pressure" and xue means "the cavities." Dian xue refers to those qin na techniques that specialize in attacking acupuncture cavities to immobilize or kill an opponent.

**dian xue an mo.** A Chinese massage technique in which the acupuncture cavities are stimulated through pressing. Dian xue massage is also called acupressure and is the root of Japanese shiatsu.

**du mai.** Usually translated as "governing vessel." One of the eight extraordinary vessels.

**Gao, Tao.** Master Yang, Jwing-Ming's first taijiquan master.

**gong (kung).** Energy or hard work.

**gongfu (kung fu).** Literally, "energy-time." Any study, learning, or practice that requires a lot of patience, energy, and time to complete. Because practicing Chinese martial arts requires a great deal of time and energy, Chinese martial arts are commonly called gongfu.

**Guoshu.** Abbreviation of "Zhongguo wushu," which means "Chinese martial techniques."

**Han, Ching-Tang.** A well-known Chinese martial artist (especially in Taiwan) in the last forty years. Master Han is also Dr. Yang, Jwing-Ming's Long Fist grand master.

**he.** Harmony or peace.

**huantiao (GB-30).** An acupuncture point that belongs to the gall bladder primary qi channel.

**huiyin (Co-1).** An acupuncture cavity belonging to the conception vessel.

**jianjing (GB-21).** An acupuncture cavity belonging to the gall bladder primary qi channel.

**jiexi (S-41).** An acupuncture cavity belonging to the stomach primary qi channel.

**jin.** Means "tendons."

**Jin, Shao-Feng.** Dr. Yang, Jwing-Ming's White Crane grand master.

**jing.** Essence. The most refined part of anything.

**jing.** Calm and silent.

**jing.** Channels. Sometimes translated "meridians." They refer to the twelve organ-related "rivers" that circulate qi throughout the body.

**juliao (GB-29).** An acupuncture cavity belonging to the gall bladder primary qi channel.

**karate.** Literally, "bare hand." Karate do is the "bare-hand way." A Japanese martial art rooted in Chinese Southern White Crane.

**kung (gong).** Means "energy" or "hard work."

**kung fu (gongfu).** Literally, "energy-time." Any study, learning, or practice that requires a lot of patience, energy, and time to complete. Because practicing Chinese martial arts requires a great deal of time and energy, Chinese martial arts are commonly called kung fu.

**Kuoshu (Guoshu).** Literally, "national techniques." Another name for Chinese martial arts. First used by President Chiang, Kai-Shek in 1928 at the founding of the Nanking Central Guoshu Institute.

**laogong (P-8).** Name of a cavity on the pericardium channel in the center of the palm.

**Li, Mao-Ching.** Dr. Yang, Jwing-Ming's Long Fist master.

**lingtai (Gv-10).** An acupuncture cavity belonging to the governing vessel.

**luo.** The small qi channels that branch out from the primary qi channels and are connected to the skin and to the bone marrow.

**mai.** Means "vessel" or "qi channel."

**mian.** Soft.

**mingmen (Gv-4).** Name of an acupuncture cavity belonging to the governing vessel.

**na.** Means "to hold" or "to grab."

**nei dan.** Literally, "internal elixir." A form of qigong in which qi (the elixir) is built up in the body and spread out to the limbs.

**nei shi fan ting.** Means "to see internally and to listen inwardly."

**nei shi gongfu.** Nei shi means "to look internally," so nei shi gongfu refers to the art of looking inside yourself to read the state of your health and the condition of your qi.

**nei wai he yi.** Literally, "internal and external unified as one." Means the unification of the external action and the internal qi.

**nei wai xie he.** Literally, "internal and external harmonized." Means the harmonious coordination of physical action and the internal mind and qi.

**pu tong an mo.** General massage. The massage for physical and mental relaxation and enjoyment.

**qi (chi).** The general definition of qi is: universal energy, including heat, light, and electromagnetic energy. A narrower definition of qi refers to the energy circulating in human or animal bodies. A current popular model is that the qi circulating in the human body is bioelectric in nature.

**qi an mo.** Qi massage. One of the high levels of massage techniques in which a massage doctor will use his or her qi to remove the qi stagnation in a patient's body. Qi massage is also called "wai qi liao fa," which means "healing with the external qi."

**qi jing ba mai.** Literally, "strange (odd) channels eight vessels." Usually referred to as "the eight extraordinary vessels" or simply as "the vessels." Called odd or strange because they are not well understood and some of them do not exist in pairs.

**qie zhen.** Palpation. One of the diagnostic techniques used in Chinese medicine.

**qigong (chi kung).** Gong means gongfu (literally, "energy-time"). Therefore, qigong means study, research, and practices related to qi.

**qigong an mo.** Qigong massage.

**qihai (Co-6).** An acupuncture cavity belonging to the conception vessel.

**re qi.** Re means "warmth" or "heat." Generally, re qi is used to represent heat. It is used sometimes to imply that a person or animal is still alive because the body is warm.

**rou.** Rub. A common massage technique.

**ren mai.** Conception vessel. One of the eight extraordinary vessels.

**shang dan tian.** Upper dan tian. Located at the third eye, it is the residence of the shen (spirit).

**shangliao (B-31).** One of four cavities on each side of the sacrum that belongs to the bladder primary qi channel.

**Shaolin.** "Young woods." Name of the Shaolin Temple.

**Shaolin Temple.** A monastery located in Henan Province, China. The Shaolin Temple is well known because of its martial arts training.

**shen.** Spirit. According to Chinese qigong, the shen resides at the upper dan tian (shang dan tian) (the third eye).

**shenshu (B-23).** Name of an acupuncture cavity that belongs to the bladder qi channel.

**shi er jing.** The twelve primary qi channels in Chinese medicine.

**shou jue yin xin bao luo jing.** Arm absolute yin pericardium channel. One of the twelve primary qi channels.

**shou shao yang san jiao jing.** Arm lesser yang triple burner channel. One of the twelve primary qi channels.

**shou shao yin xin jing.** Arm lesser yin heart channel. One of the twelve primary qi channels.

**shou tai yang xiao chang jing.** Arm greater yang small intestine channel. One of the twelve primary qi channels.

**shou tai yin fei jing.** Arm greater yin lung channel. One of the twelve primary qi channels.

**shou yang ming da chang jing.** Arm yang brightness large intestine channel. One of the twelve primary qi channels.

**tai chi chuan (taijiquan).** A Chinese internal martial style based on the theory of taiji (grand ultimate).

**taiji.** Means "grand ultimate." It is this force that generates two poles, yin and yang.

**taijiquan (tai chi chuan).** A Chinese internal martial style based on the theory of taiji (grand ultimate).

**Taipei.** The capital city of Taiwan located in the north.

**Taiwan.** An island to the southeast of mainland China. Also known as Formosa.

**Taiwan University.** A well-known university located in northern Taiwan.

**Tamkang.** Name of a university in Taiwan.

**Tamkang College Guoshu Club.** A Chinese martial arts club founded by Dr. Yang when he was studying in Tamkang College.

**tian.** Heaven or sky. In ancient China, people believed that heaven was the most powerful natural energy in this universe.

**tian qi.** Heaven qi. It is now commonly used to mean the weather, because weather is governed by heaven qi.

**tie ban qiao.** Literally, "iron board bridge." A special martial arts strength and endurance training for the torso.

**tui.** Push. A major technique in Chinese tui na qigong massage.

**tui na.** Means "to push and grab." A category of Chinese massages for healing and injury treatment.

**wai dan.** External elixir. External qigong exercises in which a practitioner will build up the qi in his limbs and then lead it into the center of the body for nourishment.

**wai dan chi kung (wai dan qigong).** External elixir qigong. In wai dan qigong, a practitioner will generate qi to the limbs and then allow the qi to flow inward to nourish the internal organs.

**wai qi liao fa.** Literally, "external qi healing." One of the high levels of qi massage in which a doctor will use his or her qi to remove qi stagnation in the patient.

**wang zhen.** Looking. One of the diagnostic techniques used in Chinese medicine.

**wei qi.** Protective qi or guardian qi. The qi at the surface of the body that generates a shield to protect the body from negative external influences such as colds.

**weizhong (B-54).** An acupuncture cavity belonging to the bladder primary qi channel.

**wen zhen.** Asking. One of the diagnostic techniques used in Chinese medicine.

**wen zhen.** Listening and smelling. Two of the diagnostic techniques used in Chinese medicine.

**Wilson Chen.** Dr. Yang, Jwing-Ming's friend.

**wu tiao.** Five regulating methods in qigong practice that include regulating the body, regulating the breathing, regulating the mind, regulating the qi, and regulating the spirit.

**Wudang Mountain.** Located in Hubei Province in China.

**wuji.** Means "no extremity."

**wushu.** Literally, "martial techniques." A common name for the Chinese martial arts. Many other terms are used, including wuyi (martial arts), wugong (martial gongfu), guoshu (national techniques), and gongfu (energy-time). Because wushu has been modified in mainland China over the past forty years into gymnastic martial performance, many traditional Chinese martial artists have given up this name in order to avoid confusing modern wushu with traditional wushu. Recently, mainland China has attempted to bring modern wushu back toward its traditional training and practice.

**xia dan tian.** Lower dan tian. Located in the lower abdomen, it is believed to be the residence of water qi (original qi).

**xialiao (B-34).** One of four cavities on each side of the sacrum that belongs to bladder primary qi channel.

**xian gu.** Means "immortal bone." The sacrum is called immortal bone in Daoist qigong practice.

**xiao.** Filial piety.

**xin.** Means "heart." Xin means the mind generated from emotional disturbance.

**xin.** Trust.

**xin xi xiang yi.** "Heart (mind) and breathing (are) mutually dependent."

**Xinzhu Xian.** Birthplace of Dr. Yang, Jwing-Ming in Taiwan.

**yang.** In Chinese philosophy, the active, positive, masculine polarity. In Chinese medicine, yang means excessive, overactive, overheated. The yang organs are the gall bladder, small intestine, large intestine, stomach, bladder, and triple burner.

**Yang, Jwing-Ming.** Author of this book.

**yangchiao mai.** Yang heel vessel. One of the eight qi vessels.

**yanglingquan (GB-34).** An acupuncture cavity belonging to the gall bladder primary qi channel.

**yangwei mai.** Yang Linking vessel. One of the eight vessels.

**yaobeitengtong.** Means "pain in the back and loin"; lumbago and back pain. Chinese medical terminology.

**yaojitong.** Means "pain along the spinal column." Chinese medical terminology.

**yaokaotong.** Means "lumbosacral pain." Chinese medical terminology.

**yaosuan.** Means "soreness of waist." Chinese medical terminology.

**yaotong.** Means "lumbago." Chinese medical terminology.

**yi.** Mind. Specifically, the mind that is generated by clear thinking and judgment and that is able to make you calm, peaceful, and wise.

**yi shen yu qi.** Use the shen (spirit) to govern the qi. A qigong technique. Because the shen is the headquarters for the qi, it is the most effective way to control it.

**yi shou dan tian.** "Keep your yi on your lower dan tian." In qigong training, you keep your mind at the lower dan tian in order to build up qi. When you are circulating your qi, you always lead your qi back to your lower dan tian before you stop.

**yi yi yin qi.** "Use your yi (wisdom mind) to lead your qi." A qigong technique. Yi cannot be pushed, but it can be led. This is best done with the yi.

**yin.** In Chinese philosophy, the passive, negative, feminine polarity. In Chinese medicine, yin means deficient. The yin organs are the heart, lungs, liver, kidneys, spleen, and pericardium.

**yinchiao mai.** The yin heel vessel. One of the eight vessels.

**yinwei mai.** Yin linking vessel. One of the eight vessels.

**yongquan (K-1).** Bubbling well. Name of an acupuncture cavity belonging to the kidney primary qi channel.

**yuan jing.** Original essence. The fundamental, original substance inherited from your parents, it is converted into original qi.

**yuan qi.** Original qi. The qi created from the original essence inherited from your parents.

**zhen dan tian.** The real dan tian, which is located at the physical center of gravity.

**zhibian (B-49).** An acupuncture cavity belonging to the bladder primary qi channel.

**zhong dan tian.** Middle dan tian. Located in the area of the solar plexus, it is the residence of fire qi.

**zhongliao (B-33).** One of four cavities on each side of the sacrum that belongs to the bladder primary qi channel.

**zu jue yin gan jing.** Leg absolute yin liver channel. One of the twelve primary qi channels.

**zu shao yang dan jing.** Leg lesser yang gall bladder channel. One of the twelve primary qi channels.

**zu shao yin shen jing.** Leg lesser yin kidney channel. One of the twelve primary qi channels.

**zu tai yang pang guang jing.** Leg greater yang bladder channel. One of the twelve primary qi channels.

**zu tai yin pi jing.** Leg greater yin spleen channel. One of the twelve primary qi channels.

**zu yang ming wei jing.** Leg yang brightness stomach channel. One of the twelve primary qi channels.

**zusanli (S-36).** An acupuncture cavity belonging to the stomach primary qi channel.

# About the Author

## Yang, Jwing-Ming, PhD (楊俊敏博士)

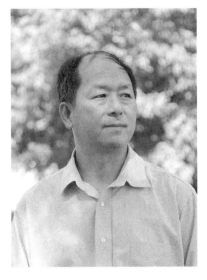

Dr. Yang, Jwing-Ming was born on August 11, 1946, in Xinzhu Xian, Taiwan, Republic of China. He started his wushu (gongfu or kung fu) training at the age of fifteen under Shaolin White Crane (Shaolin Bai He) Master Cheng, Gin-Gsao (曾金灶). Master Cheng originally learned taizuquan from his grandfather when he was a child. When Master Cheng was fifteen years old, he started learning White Crane from Master Jin, Shao-Feng (金紹峰) and followed him for twenty-three years until Master Jin's death.

In thirteen years of study (1961–1974) under Master Cheng, Dr. Yang became an expert in the White Crane style of Chinese martial arts, which includes both the use of bare hands and various weapons, such as saber, staff, spear, trident, two short rods, and many others. With the same master, he also studied White Crane qigong, qin na (chin na), tui na, and dian xue massages and herbal treatment.

At sixteen, Dr. Yang began the study of Yang-style taijiquan under Master Kao Tao (高濤). He later continued his study of taijiquan under Master Li, Mao-Ching (李茂清) and was also a student with Mr. Wilson Chen (陳威伸) in Taipei. Master Li learned his taijiquan from the well-known Master Han, Ching-Tang (韓慶堂), and Mr. Chen learned his taijiquan from Master Chang, Xiang-San (張詳三). From this further practice, Dr. Yang was able to master the taiji bare-hand sequence, pushing hands, the two-man fighting sequence, taiji sword, taiji saber, and taiji qigong.

When Dr. Yang was eighteen years old, he entered Tamkang College in Taipei Xian to study physics. In college, he began the study of traditional Shaolin Long Fist (changquan or chang chuan) with Master Li, Mao-Ching at the Tamkang College Guoshu Club, 1964–1968, and eventually became an assistant instructor under Master Li. In 1971 he completed his MS degree in physics at the National Taiwan University and then served in the Chinese Air Force from 1971 to 1972. In the service, Dr. Yang taught physics at the Junior Academy of the Chinese Air Force while also teaching wushu. After being honorably discharged in 1972, he returned to Tamkang College to teach physics and resumed study under Master Li, Mao-Ching. From Master Li, Dr. Yang learned Northern-style wushu, which includes bare-hand and kicking techniques as well as numerous weapons.

In 1974 Dr. Yang came to the United States to study mechanical engineering at Purdue University. At the request of a few students, Dr. Yang began to teach gongfu (kung fu), which resulted in the establishment of the Purdue University Chinese Kung Fu Research Club in the spring of 1975. While at Purdue, Dr. Yang also taught college-credit courses in taijiquan. In May 1978, he was awarded a PhD in mechanical engineering by Purdue.

In 1980 Dr. Yang moved to Houston to work for Texas Instruments. While in Houston, he founded Yang's Shaolin Kung Fu Academy, which was eventually taken over by his disciple, Mr. Jeffery Bolt, after Dr. Yang moved to Boston in 1982. Dr. Yang founded Yang's Martial Arts Academy in Boston on October 1, 1982.

In January 1984, he gave up his engineering career to devote more time to research, writing, and teaching. In March 1986, he purchased property in the Jamaica Plain area of Boston to be used as the headquarters of the new organization, Yang's Martial Arts Association (YMAA). The organization expanded to become a division of Yang's Oriental Arts Association, Inc. (YOAA).

In 2008 Dr. Yang began the nonprofit YMAA California Retreat Center. This training facility in rural California is where selected students enroll in a five-year residency to learn Chinese martial arts.

Dr. Yang has been involved in traditional Chinese wushu since 1961, studying Shaolin White Crane (bai he), Shaolin Long Fist (changquan), and taijiquan under several different masters. He has taught for almost fifty years: seven years in Taiwan, five years at Purdue University, two years in Houston, twenty-six years in Boston, and more than eight years at the YMAA California Retreat Center. He has taught seminars all over the world, sharing his knowledge of Chinese martial arts and qigong in Argentina, Austria, Barbados, Botswana, Belgium, Bermuda, Brazil, Canada, China, Chile, England, Egypt, France, Germany, Hungary, Iceland, Iran, Ireland, Italy, Latvia, Mexico, the Netherlands, New Zealand, Poland, Portugal, Saudi Arabia, South Africa, Spain, Switzerland, and Venezuela.

Since 1986 YMAA has become an international organization, which currently includes more than fifty schools located in Argentina, Belgium, Canada, Chile, France, Hungary, Iran, Ireland, Italy, New Zealand, Poland, Portugal, South Africa, Sweden, the United Kingdom, the United States, and Venezuela.

Many of Dr. Yang's books and videos have been translated into other languages, such as French, Italian, Spanish, Polish, Czech, Bulgarian, Russian, German, and Hungarian.

# Books and Videos by Dr. Yang, Jwing-Ming

## Books Alphabetical

*Analysis of Shaolin Chin Na*, 2nd ed. YMAA Publication Center, 1987, 2004

*Ancient Chinese Weapons: A Martial Artist's Guide*, 2nd ed. YMAA Publication Center, 1985, 1999

*Arthritis Relief: Chinese Qigong for Healing & Prevention*, 2nd ed. YMAA Publication Center, 1991, 2005

*Back Pain Relief: Chinese Qigong for Healing and Prevention*, 2nd ed. YMAA Publication Center, 1997, 2004

*Baguazhang: Theory and Applications*, 2nd ed. YMAA Publication Center, 1994, 2008

*Comprehensive Applications of Shaolin Chin Na: The Practical Defense of Chinese Seizing Arts*. YMAA Publication Center, 1995

*Essence of Shaolin White Crane*. YMAA Publication Center, 1996

*How to Defend Yourself*. YMAA Publication Center, 1992

*Introduction to Ancient Chinese Weapons*. Unique Publications, Inc., 1985

*Meridian Qigong*, YMAA Publication Center, 2016

*Northern Shaolin Sword*, 2nd ed. YMAA Publication Center, 1985, 2000

*Qigong for Health and Martial Arts*, 2nd ed. YMAA Publication Center, 1995, 1998

*Qigong Massage: Fundamental Techniques for Health and Relaxation*, 2nd ed. YMAA Publication Center, 1992, 2005

*Qigong Meditation: Embryonic Breathing*. YMAA Publication Center, 2003

*Qigong Meditation: Small Circulation*. YMAA Publication Center, 2006

*Qigong, the Secret of Youth: Da Mo's Muscle/Tendon Changing and Marrow/Brain Washing Qigong*, 2nd ed. YMAA Publication Center, 1989, 2000

*Root of Chinese Qigong: Secrets of Qigong Training*, 2nd ed. YMAA Publication Center, 1989, 2004

*Shaolin Chin Na*. Unique Publications, Inc., 1980

*Shaolin Long Fist Kung Fu*. Unique Publications, Inc., 1981

*Simple Qigong Exercises for Health: The Eight Pieces of Brocade*, 3rd ed. YMAA Publication Center, 1988, 1997, 2013

*Tai Chi Ball Qigong: For Health and Martial Arts*. YMAA Publication Center, 2010

*Tai Chi Chin Na: The Seizing Art of Taijiquan*, 2nd ed. YMAA Publication Center, 1995, 2014

*Tai Chi Chuan Classical Yang Style: The Complete Long Form and Qigong*, 2nd ed. YMAA Publication Center, 1999, 2010

*Tai Chi Chuan Martial Applications*, 2nd ed. YMAA Publication Center, 1986, 1996

*Tai Chi Chuan Martial Power*, 3rd ed. YMAA Publication Center, 1986, 1996, 2015

*Tai Chi Chuan: Classical Yang Style*, 2nd ed. YMAA Publication Center, 1999, 2010

*Tai Chi Qigong: The Internal Foundation of Tai Chi Chuan*, 2nd ed. rev. YMAA Publication Center, 1997, 1990, 2013

*Tai Chi Secrets of the Ancient Masters: Selected Readings with Commentary*. YMAA Publication Center, 1999

*Tai Chi Secrets of the Wû and Li Styles: Chinese Classics, Translation, Commentary*. YMAA Publication Center, 2001

*Tai Chi Secrets of the Wu Style: Chinese Classics, Translation, Commentary*. YMAA Publication Center, 2002

*Tai Chi Secrets of the Yang Style: Chinese Classics, Translation, Commentary*. YMAA Publication Center, 2001

*Tai Chi Sword Classical Yang Style: The Complete Long Form, Qigong, and Applications*, 2nd ed. YMAA Publication Center, 1999, 2014

*Taijiquan Theory of Dr. Yang, Jwing-Ming: The Root of Taijiquan*. YMAA Publication Center, 2003

*Xingyiquan: Theory and Applications*, 2nd ed. YMAA Publication Center, 1990, 2003

*Yang Style Tai Chi Chuan.* Unique Publications, Inc., 1981

## Videos Alphabetical

*Advanced Practical Chin Na in Depth.* YMAA Publication Center, 2010

*Analysis of Shaolin Chin Na.* YMAA Publication Center, 2004

*Baguazhang (Eight Trigrams Palm Kung Fu).* YMAA Publication Center, 2005

*Chin Na in Depth: Courses 1-4.* YMAA Publication Center, 2003

*Chin Na in Depth: Courses 5-8.* YMAA Publication Center, 2003

*Chin Na in Depth: Courses 9-12.* YMAA Publication Center, 2003

*Five Animal Sports Qigong.* YMAA Publication Center, 2008

*Knife Defense: Traditional Techniques.* YMAA Publication Center, 2011

*Meridian Qigong.* YMAA Publication Center, 2015

*Neigong.* YMAA Publication Center, 2015

*Northern Shaolin Sword.* YMAA Publication Center, 2009

*Qigong Massage.* YMAA Publication Center, 2005

*Saber Fundamental Training.* YMAA Publication Center, 2008

*Shaolin Kung Fu Fundamental Training.* YMAA Publication Center, 2004

*Shaolin Long Fist Kung Fu: Basic Sequences.* YMAA Publication Center, 2005

*Shaolin Saber Basic Sequences.* YMAA Publication Center, 2007

*Shaolin Staff Basic Sequences.* YMAA Publication Center, 2007

*Shaolin White Crane Gong Fu Basic Training: Courses 1 & 2.* YMAA Publication Center, 2003

*Shaolin White Crane Gong Fu Basic Training: Courses 3 & 4.* YMAA Publication Center, 2008

*Shaolin White Crane Hard and Soft Qigong.* YMAA Publication Center, 2003

*Shuai Jiao: Kung Fu Wrestling.* YMAA Publication Center, 2010

*Simple Qigong Exercises for Arthritis Relief.* YMAA Publication Center, 2007

*Simple Qigong Exercises for Back Pain Relief.* YMAA Publication Center, 2007

*Simple Qigong Exercises for Health: The Eight Pieces of Brocade.* YMAA Publication Center, 2003

*Staff Fundamental Training: Solo Drills and Matching Practice.* YMAA Publication Center, 2007

*Sword Fundamental Training.* YMAA Publication Center, 2009

*Tai Chi Ball Qigong: Courses 1 & 2.* YMAA Publication Center, 2006

*Tai Chi Ball Qigong: Courses 3 & 4.* YMAA Publication Center, 2007

*Tai Chi Chuan: Classical Yang Style.* YMAA Publication Center, 2003

*Tai Chi Fighting Set: 2-Person Matching Set.* YMAA Publication Center, 2006

*Tai Chi Pushing Hands: Courses 1 & 2.* YMAA Publication Center, 2005

*Tai Chi Pushing Hands: Courses 3 & 4.* YMAA Publication Center, 2006

*Tai Chi Qigong.* YMAA Publication Center, 2005

*Tai Chi Sword, Classical Yang Style.* YMAA Publication Center, 2005

*Tai Chi Symbol: Yin/Yang Sticking Hands.* YMAA Publication Center, 2008

*Taiji 37 Postures Martial Applications.* YMAA Publication Center, 2008

*Taiji Chin Na in Depth.* YMAA Publication Center, 2009

*Taiji Saber: Classical Yang Style.* YMAA Publication Center, 2008

*Taiji Wrestling: Advanced Takedown Techniques.* YMAA Publication Center, 2008

*Understanding Qigong, DVD 1: What Is Qigong? The Human Qi Circulatory System.* YMAA Publication Center, 2006

*Understanding Qigong, DVD 2: Key Points of Qigong & Qigong Breathing.* YMAA Publication Center, 2006

*Understanding Qigong, DVD 3: Embryonic Breathing.* YMAA Publication Center, 2007

*Understanding Qigong, DVD 4: Four Seasons Qigong.* YMAA Publication Center, 2007

*Understanding Qigong, DVD 5: Small Circulation.* YMAA Publication Center, 2007

*Understanding Qigong, DVD 6: Martial Arts Qigong Breathing.* YMAA Publication Center, 2007

*Xingyiquan: Twelve Animals Kung Fu and Applications.* YMAA Publication Center, 2008

*Yang Tai Chi for Beginners.* YMAA Publication Center, 2012

*YMAA 25-Year Anniversary.* YMAA Publication Center, 2009

# Index

**Westfield Memorial Library**
**Westfield, New Jersey**

**Westfield Memorial Library**
**Westfield, New Jersey**

**Westfield Memorial Library**
**Westfield, New Jersey**

# BOOKS FROM YMAA

**Westfield Memorial Library**
**Westfield, New Jersey**

## DVDS FROM YMAA

ADVANCED PRACTICAL CHIN NA IN-DEPTH

ANALYSIS OF SHAOLIN CHIN NA

ATTACK THE ATTACK

BAGUAZHANG: EMEI BAGUAZHANG

BEGINNER QIGONG FOR WOMEN

CHEN STYLE TAIJIQUAN

CHIN NA IN-DEPTH COURSES 1—4

CHIN NA IN-DEPTH COURSES 5—8

CHIN NA IN-DEPTH COURSES 9—12

FACING VIOLENCE: 7 THINGS A MARTIAL ARTIST MUST KNOW

FIVE ANIMAL SPORTS

JOINT LOCKS

KNIFE DEFENSE: TRADITIONAL TECHNIQUES AGAINST A DAGGER

KUNG FU BODY CONDITIONING 1

KUNG FU BODY CONDITIONING 2

KUNG FU FOR KIDS

KUNG FU FOR TEENS

INFIGHTING

LOGIC OF VIOLENCE

MERIDIAN QIGONG

NEIGONG FOR MARTIAL ARTS

NORTHERN SHAOLIN SWORD : SAN CAI JIAN, KUN WU JIAN, QI MEN JIAN

QIGONG MASSAGE

QIGONG FOR CANCER

QIGONG FOR HEALING

QIGONG FOR LONGEVITY

QIGONG FOR WOMEN

SABER FUNDAMENTAL TRAINING

SAI TRAINING AND SEQUENCES

SANCHIN KATA: TRADITIONAL TRAINING FOR KARATE POWER

SHAOLIN KUNG FU FUNDAMENTAL TRAINING: COURSES 1 & 2

SHAOLIN LONG FIST KUNG FU: BASIC SEQUENCES

SHAOLIN LONG FIST KUNG FU: INTERMEDIATE SEQUENCES

SHAOLIN LONG FIST KUNG FU: ADVANCED SEQUENCES 1

SHAOLIN LONG FIST KUNG FU: ADVANCED SEQUENCES 2

SHAOLIN SABER: BASIC SEQUENCES

SHAOLIN STAFF: BASIC SEQUENCES

SHAOLIN WHITE CRANE GONG FU BASIC TRAINING: COURSES 1 & 2

SHAOLIN WHITE CRANE GONG FU BASIC TRAINING: COURSES 3 & 4

SHUAI JIAO: KUNG FU WRESTLING

SIMPLE QIGONG EXERCISES FOR ARTHRITIS RELIEF

SIMPLE QIGONG EXERCISES FOR BACK PAIN RELIEF

SIMPLIFIED TAI CHI CHUAN: 24 & 48 POSTURES

SIMPLIFIED TAI CHI FOR BEGINNERS 48

SUNRISE TAI CHI

SUNSET TAI CHI

SWORD: FUNDAMENTAL TRAINING

TAEKWONDO KORYO POOMSAE

TAI CHI BALL QIGONG: COURSES 1 & 2

TAI CHI BALL QIGONG: COURSES 3 & 4

TAI CHI BALL WORKOUT FOR BEGINNERS

TAI CHI CHUAN CLASSICAL YANG STYLE

TAI CHI CONNECTIONS

TAI CHI ENERGY PATTERNS

TAI CHI FIGHTING SET

TAI CHI FIT FLOW

TAI CHI FIT OVER 50

TAI CHI FIT STRENGTH

TAI CHI FIT TO GO

TAI CHI FOR WOMEN

TAI CHI PUSHING HANDS: COURSES 1 & 2

TAI CHI PUSHING HANDS: COURSES 3 & 4

TAI CHI SWORD: CLASSICAL YANG STYLE

TAI CHI SWORD FOR BEGINNERS

TAI CHI SYMBOL: YIN YANG STICKING HANDS

TAIJI & SHAOLIN STAFF: FUNDAMENTAL TRAINING

TAIJI CHIN NA IN-DEPTH

TAIJI 37 POSTURES MARTIAL APPLICATIONS

TAIJI SABER CLASSICAL YANG STYLE

TAIJI WRESTLING

TRAINING FOR SUDDEN VIOLENCE

UNDERSTANDING QIGONG 1: WHAT IS QI? • HUMAN QI CIRCULATORY SYSTEM

UNDERSTANDING QIGONG 2: KEY POINTS • QIGONG BREATHING

UNDERSTANDING QIGONG 3: EMBRYONIC BREATHING

UNDERSTANDING QIGONG 4: FOUR SEASONS QIGONG

UNDERSTANDING QIGONG 5: SMALL CIRCULATION

UNDERSTANDING QIGONG 6: MARTIAL QIGONG BREATHING

WHITE CRANE HARD & SOFT QIGONG

WUDANG KUNG FU: FUNDAMENTAL TRAINING

WUDANG SWORD

WUDANG TAIJIQUAN

XINGYIQUAN

YANG TAI CHI FOR BEGINNERS

*more products available from . . .*

**YMAA Publication Center, Inc.** 楊氏東方文化出版中心

1-800-669-8892 • info@ymaa.com • www.ymaa.com

Westland Memorial Library
Westland, New Jersey

WESTFIELD MEMORIAL LIBRARY

3 9550 00539 6832

Westfield Memorial Library
Westfield, New Jersey

10/17

617.564 Yan
Yang, Jwing-Ming, 1946- author.
The pain-free back